FAT FRUMPY & OVER 50

3 STEPS TO FINALLY
STOP SABOTAGING YOUR WEIGHT
(& FEEL FABULOUS AGAIN)

JACQUELINE LAPTON

First Printing: 2022

Copyright © 2022 by Jacqueline Lapton

All rights reserved.

Published in Australia.

This book or any of its parts may not be reproduced or used in any manner whatsoever without the express written permission of the author and publisher. However, brief quotations in a book review or scholarly journal are permitted.

Authors and their publications mentioned in this book have their copyright protection. All brand and product names used in this book are trademarks, registered trademarks, or trade names and belong to the respective owners.

Neither the publisher nor the author is engaged in rendering professional advice or services for individual reader's health care needs that may require medical supervision. The ideas and suggestions contained in this book are not intended as a substitute for consulting a medical or other professional in matters relating to health, especially if you have existing medical conditions.

For fabulous women everywhere

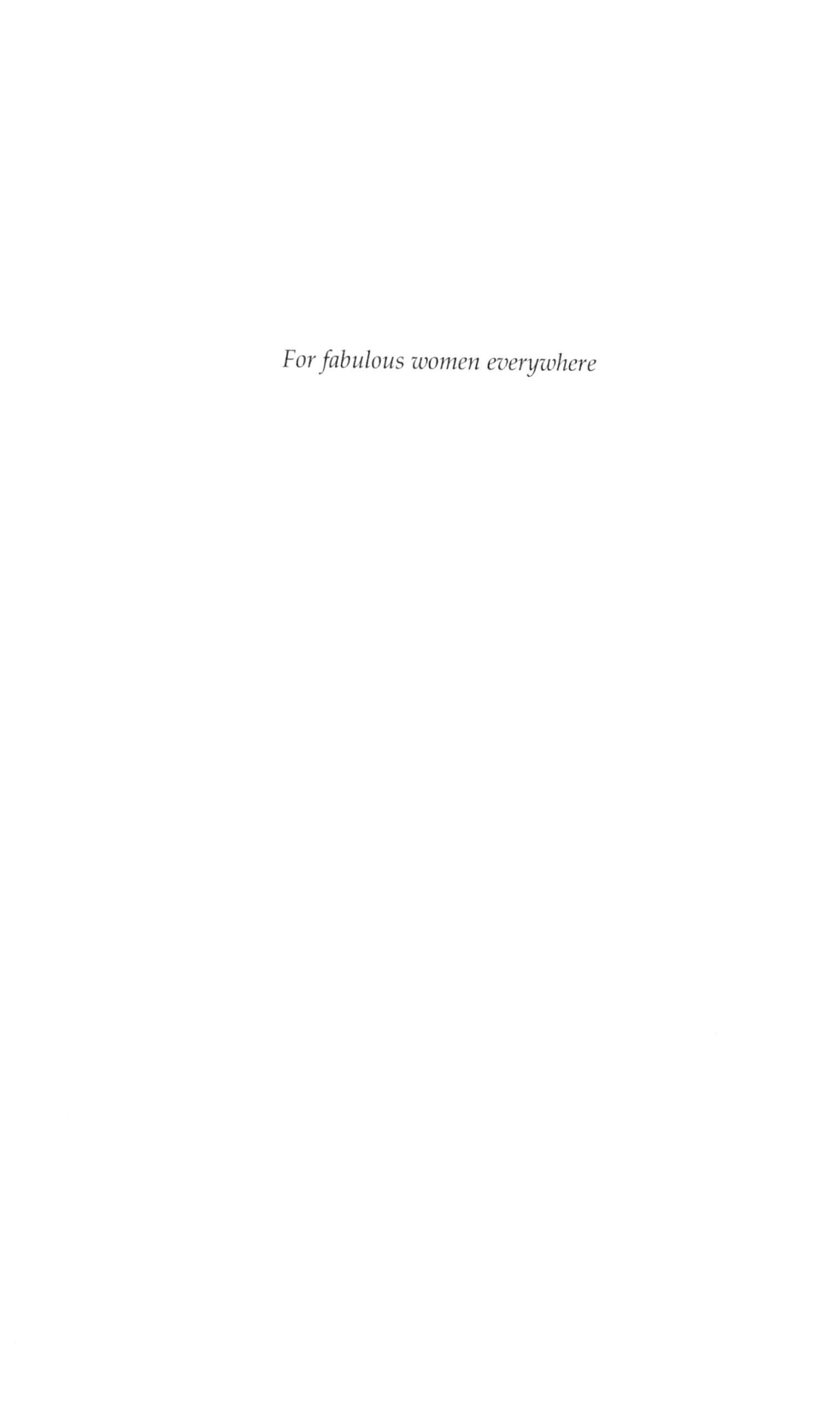

Contents

Acknowledgements	ix
About This Book	11
Step 1: Reality Check (Scare Yourself Sh**less)	13
It's a beautiful life and yet you aren't living it	14
Your present self versus your future self	16
Skating on thin ice	17
Time and tide wait for no (wo)man	19
You always have the potential to start over	20
What will be your 'a-ha' moment?	21
DIWYSC (Do It While You Still Can)	22
If not now… when?	23
Step 2: Take Control (Set Yourself Up for Success)	25
Know your 'why'	26
Start with the end in *your* mind	27
What is your current relationship with food?	29
Prepare for a major change	29
Understand the basic science of weight loss	30
Know your starting point	31
Calculate the calories you need each day	35
Lose weight but don't look older	36
Know your macronutrient requirements	37
Your week on a plate	38
Prepare your meals	39
Shapeshifters	41
Maybe you need extra support?	41
More tips for losing weight after 50	42

Step 3: Stay on Track (& Conquer Your Inner Voice)   45

   Part 1 – Prevent food cravings *before* they take hold of you   47

   Part 2 – Crush your diet-crashing cravings *in-the-moment* if they've got you in their grip   93

Conclusion   113

And One Final Thing…   115

Free Gift!

It is essential to set yourself up for success as you start out on your journey towards being a healthy weight and feeling fabulous again.

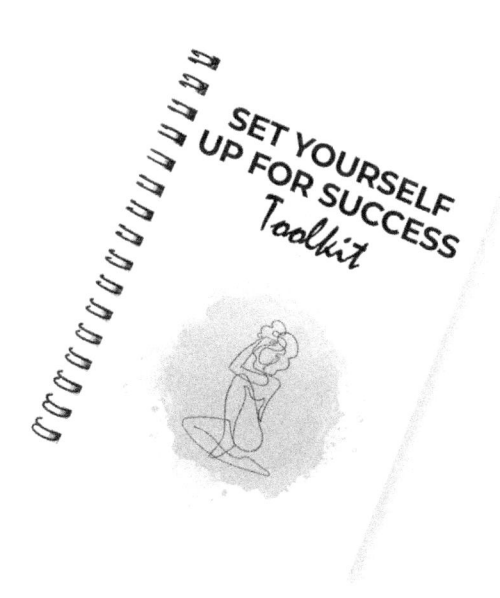

As a thank you for reading this book, and to offer you support and motivation as you go along, I would like to give you a free copy of the '**Set Yourself Up For Success Toolkit**'.

For access, email 'Free Gift' to:
freegift@fatfrumpyandover50.com

Acknowledgements

I want to give my heartfelt thanks to the amazing people who have helped me in writing this book.

Every book finds its way. And so, I am grateful to the wonderful women out there who have shared their personal journeys with me, and to their conversations and experiences that gave me purpose and momentum.

To my daughter, Georgia, an accredited practising dietitian, for her unflagging support and professional advice.

In the UK, to Christopher Payne, for his guidance and immense experience; for showing confidence in my work, and for introducing me to his telling of The Story of the Howling Dog (on page 23).

To Mohammed Musthafa for his talent in creating the cover for this book.

And to Gian Caneba for his skillful, imaginative and detailed illustrations.

Thank you all.

About This Book

Throughout your life, you have always given a lot of yourself to others… maybe raising children, supporting a business or caring for elderly parents. You have now reached a time where you are able to 'take a breather', step away and focus a bit more on yourself. In doing so, you have come face-to-face with the reality that, over the past few years, weight has been creeping on and here you are now in your 50s, overweight and feeling frumpy. And, dammit, that is not how you want to feel because you know you still have a lot more living and loving to do.

You decide it's time for action but stumble at the starting line. You are confronted with all the messages – from diet books, weight-loss programs, apps and social media – about the importance of being a healthy weight as you get older (usually to avoid poor health). But these messages fail to recognize that it's not only about being healthier, it's also about feeling fabulous again.

Most of these messages come in the form of instruction manuals 'for all ages', simply telling you what you need to do to lose weight as though it is 'flick the switch' easy. Few recognize the *challenges* of successful weight loss, especially if you're a woman in her 50s.

'Fat, Frumpy & Over 50' is different. It is a directly helpful book written for women 'mid-lifers'. It doesn't just give you instructions then say "get on with it". Instead, it recognizes that successful weight loss comes down to what goes on in the six inches between your ears. It therefore offers practical tools and strategies, in three steps, to get you into the right mindset. It will then keep you there so you can actually cross the finish line this time.

This book is *not* about a new diet to try and fail. Rather, it is an approach that will empower you to consistently make food choices that align with what matters most to you. It is based on principles, not on trends, and offers you a new way to stop sabotaging your weight over and over again.

As you have a busy life, and to support you along the way, this book is condensed and easy to read. It gives you realistic information specific to your different eating struggles. It assists you with over 100 effective everyday strategies and tools to use if you are tempted to give up again. You can simply find the ones that work best for you.

If you have the willingness to finally achieve your healthy weight goals, and to feel fabulous again, this three-step 'toolkit' will empower you to stay in control, motivated, and on track to be successful this one last time.

Step 1 is an 'in-your-face' reality check about the risks of staying overweight in your 50s, what you're missing out on in your life, and why you have to take action now.

Step 2 guides you in preparing for, and taking control of, your weight-loss journey.

Step 3 gives you all the practical tips, tools and strategies you will need to never, ever, ever give up again.

Step 1: Reality Check
(Scare Yourself Sh**less)

*Remember how long you've been putting this off,
how many extensions the gods gave you,
and you didn't use them. At some point you have
to recognize what world it is that you belong to;
what power rules it and from what source
you spring; that there is a limit to the time assigned
to you, and if you don't use it to free yourself
it will be gone and will never return.*
Marcus Aurelius

As you grow older, you can feel the whoosh of time as it rushes by you. And, too often, as you are confronted with the passage of another anniversary or birthday, you are hit with that overwhelming sadness that you haven't achieved the things you've wanted the most. You experience, yet again, that sense of melancholy and disappointment that life is speeding by too fast, and leaving you far behind.

The fact is, time seems to pass by faster because you haven't taken action towards achieving your goals. The trick to 'slowing down time' is to make *meaningful* and *consistent* progress towards achieving them and, in so doing, creating *memorable* time stamps in your daily life.

So, before more time is lost to you:
- Face up to the risks of staying overweight in your 50s, and why standing on the sidelines of your life is *no longer* an option, and
- Decide why you have to take action *now*.

✓ It's a beautiful life… and yet you aren't living it

> *While the experience of dismissal affects women of all ages, it can be magnified for those over 50. We simply stop seeing women, because we value women still for their appearance and their reproductive abilities. Once women reach menopause, we think they're past their use-by date.*
> **Jane Caro**

Have you thought "I can't believe this is happening to me? I'm turning 50 (or thereabouts) this year!"

If asked "How are you?", chances are you would say, "I'm fine", but are you really?

Being overweight can impact your self-esteem. In Western society, rightly or wrongly, there can be societal pressure to be thinner, carrying with it a negative moral value to being overweight.

Maybe you will never think of yourself as old (and at 50-something, you aren't), but being fat and frumpy makes you *feel* unattractive and probably look at least 10 years older than your years… remember that shock when you caught an unguarded glimpse of yourself in the shop window and wondered who that 'old woman' is, only to realize it's you?

When you stop and have a long look at yourself, do you see someone who has stepped back from life?

How long has it been since you could wear anything stylish? Are you always limited to shapeless, loose-fitting, monotone-colored clothes, with lots of three-quarter length sleeves (got to keep those arms covered) and *never* any horizontal stripes?

Do you even think of yourself as a sexual person anymore, or nowadays are you feeling more like a roommate with your partner?

Or maybe, just maybe, you sometimes dream of getting back into the dating game again (and possibly even great sex and an awesome relationship?).

> *It has been identified that obesity [a body mass index (BMI) > 30.0] is a significant predictor for poor psychological wellbeing and negative quality of life for women during their transition through, and post, menopause. These women tend to accumulate more body weight and this has particularly impacted physical functioning, energy and vitality, and health perceptions.*
> **Quality of life in obese postmenopausal women, G L Jones, A Sutton; Menopause International 2008**

- In the US, three in four women aged 55-64 years (74%) are overweight or obese. ('Prevalence of over weight, obesity and severe obesity among adults aged 20 and over: United States 1960-1962 through 2017-2018', Centers for Disease Control & Prevention)
- In the UK, the average BMI for women aged 55-64 years is 28.3 (in the overweight range). ('Health Survey for England', NHS, 2019)
- In Australia, two in three women aged 55-64 years (66%) are overweight or obese. ('National Health Survey 2017-18', Australian Bureau of Statistics)

✓ Your present self versus your future self

Although you absolutely believe you will get around to losing your excess weight, what if I told you that *10 years from now* this hasn't happened and you are still overweight? In fact, your weight is *exactly the same as it is today*. How would you feel? Chances are you'd be less than impressed with the decisions you continued to make throughout those years, just to end up changing nothing and being exactly where you are right now.

At every stage of your life, you have made the decisions that have profoundly influenced the person you have become. Looking backwards from today to where you were 10 years ago, I predict that at that time you truly believed your future weight would be very different, and that you always saw your future self as being fit and fabulous.

> *Your future self is watching you right now through your memories.*
> **Aubrey de Grey**

Why do you keep making decisions that your future self is so likely to regret?

One of the reasons is that you have a fundamental misconception about the power of time.

Another is that, here and now, your future self is considered a stranger who you are willing to continue to harm in favor of your present self.

Your intentions are always good, sort of… you are steadfastly 'future focused' in that you absolutely intend to start losing that excess weight again 'next Monday', you just have to get through until after your daughter's wedding or your sister's

Step 1: Reality Check (& Scare Yourself Sh**less)

birthday party, or just get [fill in the blank] done, and then you'll be ready to start. Yes, that old bandwagon. And how has that worked out for you so far?

In reality, how many Mondays have come and gone? How many times have you decided "that's a future me problem"?

No doubt, yet again, you are forgetting about all your past failed attempts. And somehow, regardless of these failures and almost magically, you still truly believe that your future weight will actually be different.

The thing is, you have chosen to be the weight you are right now. And it is not going to change by itself. *It is up to you.*

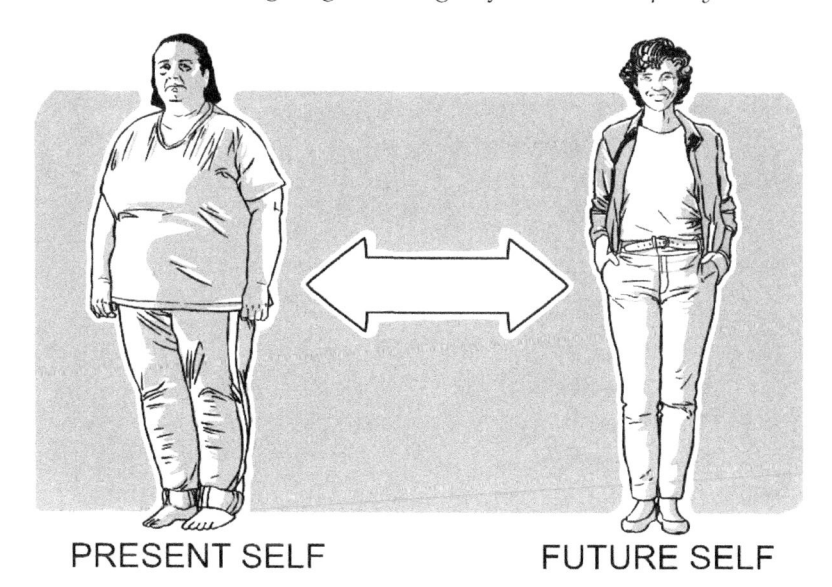

PRESENT SELF   FUTURE SELF

If only all it took was hope and wishful thinking

✅ Skating on thin ice

It's a fact that weight gain is all too common for women over the age of 50. Unfortunately, however, being overweight isn't

Fat, Frumpy & Over 50

just a vanity issue – it can also have serious, life-changing consequences.

Sure, you want to lose weight so you don't feel frumpy anymore, but it's also about your wellbeing – you want to have as many fit, active and healthy years ahead of you as possible.

> *Don't be a fatty in your fifties.*
> **Boris Johnson**

Once you reach the age of 50, weight gain, particularly around your stomach (with more visceral fat – the bad fat – around your organs), significantly increases your risk of heart disease (and heart disease accounts for nearly half of all deaths in women over 50).

There is also the increased risk of other diseases including:
- High blood pressure
- Type 2 diabetes
- Stroke
- Pulmonary embolism
- Some cancers
- A decrease in general physical function
- Decline in cognitive abilities
- Large joint osteoarthritis
- Increased body-wide inflammation
- Sleep apnoea
- Dementia and Alzheimer's disease in later life

The thing is, you're hoping to live a long, long time. However, put simply, if you are overweight, you are more likely to die at a younger age.

But what if you don't die, and you continue to be overweight? Then you're more likely to live with chronic disease or injury. And you'll continue to feel frumpy, sitting on the sidelines of your life.

Step 1: Reality Check (& Scare Yourself Sh**less)

✓ Time and tide wait for no (wo)man

*So many of us use the expression
"better late than never".
A qualification: too late is the same as never.*
JD Boatwood

Sometimes life seems really short, and at other times it seems impossibly long. Drawing your 'Life Calendar' will help to emphasize that it's certainly *finite*. There they are, all those little boxes, fully countable, staring you in the face. These are your fleeting years and they are all you've got.

Let's say you are 55 years old now, and you think you'll live to be 90, then you're already past half-way. (You can use an online 'longevity calculator' to estimate your life expectancy.)

Once you have worked out the number of years you expect to have left, think about how many you are willing to let pass you by while being unsatisfied with how you're living them. (And remember, you never *actually* know how many years you have left on earth.)

So, create your 'Life Calendar'. Visualize your life in front of you. It's a great way to see just how temporary it is.
1. Draw 10 columns on a page, then 9 lines across (90 boxes for 90 years).
2. Shade or fill in the boxes with a cross or a dot for the years you have already lived.

Then use it for inspiration to make the most of the time you have left. While you're looking at your Life Calendar, remind yourself that those empty boxes (or years) can potentially be *whatever you want them to be*. It's your choice. Life is wide open, and this calendar is a good reminder.

You have this one glorious chance at life. Are you making the most of yours?

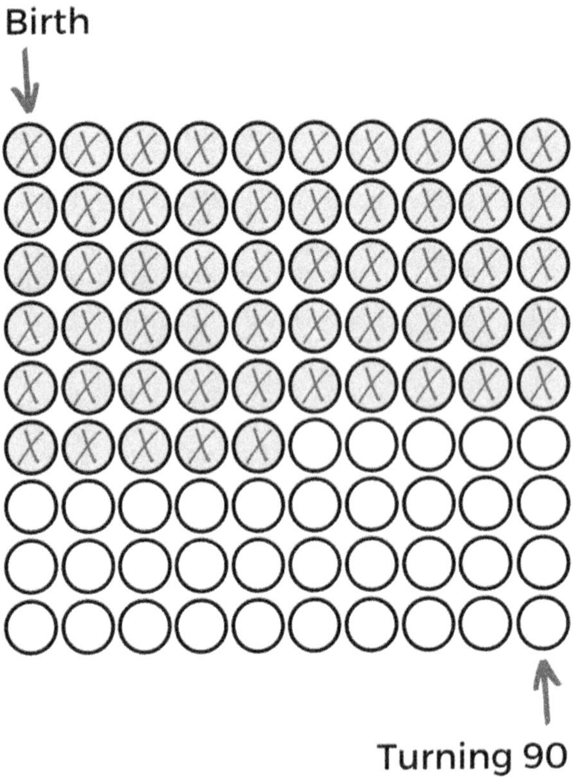
Birth
Turning 90

✓ You always have the potential to start over again

Although there are clearly downsides to reaching 'middle-age', there is also so much beauty and potential in this life stage. If you're asking yourself "Am I now too old to lose weight?", the short answer is *no*.

Although losing weight is never easy, and it can get harder after you turn 50, it is absolutely still possible. In fact, it is *never*

Step 1: Reality Check (& Scare Yourself Sh**less)

too late to start making positive changes that will impact on your weight and overall wellbeing, *unless you believe it is.*

Ask yourself, "What's the alternative?" Do nothing? Hope for the best? You already know that doesn't work.

Just because you're in your 50s, you don't have to let age define your identity and limit your belief in what is possible. Gain a new perspective and create a fresh start.

> *Though no-one can go back and make a brand-new start, anyone can start from now and make a brand-new ending.*
> **Carl Brand**

✓ What will be your 'a-ha' moment?

What will be your tipping point, the one that will motivate you to change? When will you acknowledge that you have hit rock bottom, and that you are sick and tired of being overweight and feeling frumpy?

What 'great flash of awareness' will propel you towards taking the action you need to take to have a fit and fabulous future?

Will it be a health-related diagnosis that makes you realize you're running out of time – the thought of dying can teach you a lot about living – or perhaps you don't want to be missing from any more family photos (because you refuse to hide from the camera anymore)?

Or maybe it will be something much more everyday such as seeing your photo on Facebook, or looking in the mirror and seeing your mother staring back?

'Rock bottom' is whatever you decide to make it. Decide what it is *now*.

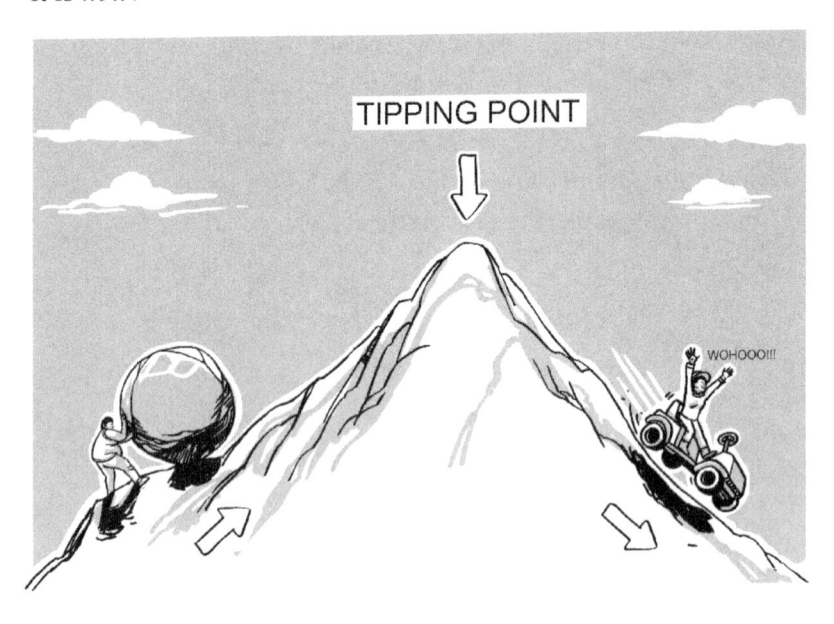

✓ DIWYST (Do It While You Still Can)

What life-changing 'crisis' will it take for you to realize that your time is limited?

Or, will you wait another 10 or more years until one day when you wake up and find there isn't any more time left to choose to get back to being a healthy weight and to feel fabulous again? That you have left it too late...

It's common to think "I'll start next week" or "I'll start after New Year", etc., etc. But the thing is, there is never going to be a 'perfect' time to start. This is just a recipe for inaction. Stop waiting for more 'Mondays' to see what happens with your life. Don't wait until things get easier, simpler, better because life will always be complicated.

Step 1: Reality Check (& Scare Yourself Sh**less)

Just start today, because you can never know, or count on, what tomorrow might bring.

The Story of the Howling Dog

A man moved into a quiet neighborhood. He went for a walk one morning, and he walked past a house. On the porch was a dog howling away. Behind the dog sat an old farmer on a rocking chair. The man asked the farmer, "Why is your dog howling?" The farmer answered, "Probably because he is sitting on a nail." The man glanced at the dog, bewildered, but then carried on walking around the block. As he came back again, he saw the dog still on the porch, howling away. Surprised, the man asked, "Well, why won't he get off?" The farmer chuckled and said, "Probably because it doesn't hurt enough yet."

✓ If not now, when?

Ask yourself, "If not now… *when*?" (Translation: Anything that is worth pursuing is worth pursuing *in this moment*.) If your answer is *now*, you will have to make a decision and accept that there are some things you will have to do for as long as it takes, and stick at no matter what, that you won't actually like doing (to start with). You will have to be strong enough to begin right now. And you will have to understand that this requires 100% commitment from you (because 99% commitment is not an option).

> *It is easier to adjust ourselves to the hardships of a poor living than it is to adjust ourselves to the hardships of making a better one. The secret of success lies in forming the habits of doing things that failures don't like to do. Success is something which is achieved by a minority of (wo)men and is therefore unnatural and not to be achieved by following our natural likes and dislikes nor by being guided by our natural preferences and prejudices... You will never succeed beyond the purpose to which you are willing to surrender.*
> **Albert E. N. Gray**
> **(The Common Denominator of Success)**

Step 2: Take Control
(& Set Yourself Up for Success)

The next step is about preparing for your weight-loss success before you start. Giving yourself a solid foundation will allow you to then focus on achieving and sustaining it.

By getting into a state of readiness you will:
- Have all the information and support tools on hand
- Feel empowered to make informed decisions and choices while moving forward
- Know your starting point so you can understand where you are right now; where you want to get to; how you're going to get there, and how well you're travelling along the way

Let's start...

> *Success is 90 percent preparation.*
> **Peter James**

✅ Know your 'why'

At this point, the most important thing is your motivation for making positive changes. Finding and connecting with your 'why', or purpose, will get you thinking about what really matters to you.

Instead of starting with the 'what', 'how' and 'when' in your life, change your approach and start with your 'why'. Then the rest will naturally follow. Starting with your 'why' will give you the foundation from which to take inspired action towards achieving your goal of being a healthy weight.

When you really understand your 'why', and it is truly important to you, your underlying motivators will kick in and get you living your best life.

To do this:
1. Write down *all* your reasons for losing weight (not just the number on the scales). Be specific.

    What is really motivating you? What are your feelings? Is it for better health? To have more energy? To feel less tired? So that it is easier to walk and move around? To lift your mood and have a positive outlook on life? To improve your self-confidence? To wear better clothes? Or simply to feel fabulous again?

    Remember that your intention can be either to avoid pain or to seek pleasure.

2. Now check that your reasons have enough 'depth' – that you are absolutely passionate about them and they are important enough to you to motivate change.

An example of a *pain-avoiding* 'why':
"I want to lose weight because I had a health scare last week

Step 2: Take Control (& Set Yourself Up for Success)

that terrified me that I would not be able to care for my elderly parents, support my daughter, or look after my dogs if I was no longer around. I felt dreadful that I would have played a role in that outcome by failing to lose weight and look after my health."

An example of a *pleasure seeking* 'why':
"I want to be alive, fit, healthy, and full of energy at each of my children's 50th birthdays, and to know I have been there as a positive, healthy role model throughout their lives."

> *Suddenly, again, a feeling, known on more than one occasion as a child, an unbearable intensification of all senses, a magical and demanding impulse, the presence of something for which it was alone worth living.*
> **Vladimir Nabokov, Glory**

✓ Start with the end in (your) mind

Goals take your 'why' and turn it into 'what', 'when' and 'how'.

When setting your goals make sure they:
- Are value-based and reflect your personal and emotional 'why'
- Excite you (otherwise they can turn into chores, and chores are easy to put off)
- Are positive – things you *can* do or have rather than things you *can't* (when it comes to losing weight, think about all the things you get to do each day rather than the things you'll be going without for a while)

- Are based on the feelings or experience you hope to get from achieving them (maybe validation, peace, intimacy, freedom, excitement, how you want to wake up feeling every day)
- Are S.M.A.R.T. (Specific, Measurable, Achievable, Realistic and anchored within a Time Frame)

The goal-setting process forces you to reflect on:
1. *What* the goal is that you want to achieve.
2. *When* you will achieve it.
3. *How* you will achieve it.
4. *Why* this goal is important to you and how you will feel after you have achieved it.

Goal Setting Worksheet
What is the goal that I want to achieve?   To lose 30 pounds (13 kilograms) and reduce my waist circumference to below 32 inches (80 centimeters).
When will I achieve this goal?   I am starting today and will reach my goal by the 1st [month] [year], 6 months from now.
How am I going to achieve this goal?   I am following a 1,600-calorie healthy meal plan.   I am walking for 30 minutes 5 days a week.
Why is this goal important to me?   *How will I feel after I have achieved it?*   I can now fit into that pair of designer jeans I've had in my wardrobe for years and I feel smart and super-stylish.

> *Success is no accident. Living an incredible life is no accident. You'll have to do it on purpose.*
> ## *Carrie Green*

✓ What is your current relationship with food?

Before you can work towards a 'good' relationship with food, understand your current relationship by asking yourself the following questions:
"Do I…
- notice that I am preoccupied with food?"
- feel guilty about eating and often eat in secret?"
- struggle to eat some foods in moderation?"
- reach for food when I am upset or stressed?"
- have a history of yo-yo dieting?"
- find myself restricting or bingeing food?"
- often eat until I am uncomfortably full?"
- make bargains with myself to eat certain foods?"
- often eat mindlessly?"

If your relationship with food is on the 'bad' side, you probably answered yes to a few, or even many, of these questions (and I imagine you're not surprised). At least, now, you can see it clearly for what it is.

Next, record everything you eat for a few days so you can identify your current eating behaviors and patterns.

✓ Prepare for a major change

Consider getting checked by a healthcare professional before you start.

A visit to your doctor can:
- Help you get a better picture of how being overweight is affecting your health and wellbeing
- Provide you with a baseline of your health status
- Rule out conditions that may be making it difficult to

lose weight even though you have been active and following a healthy diet (for example, a vitamin D deficiency can cause you to store fat faster, and make it more difficult to lose weight – you may want to ask your doctor to check your level)
- Assist you to get a referral to a dietitian

Seeing a dietitian can:
- Help you create a personalized nutrition and weight-loss plan, including weight-loss goals and ways to achieve them (this can be an advantage over a self-guided program or app)
- Provide a check-in on your progress
- Offer support and counseling if you experience road-blocks

✅ Understand the basic science of weight loss

The reason you are overweight is that you consume too many calories and don't move enough (but I suspect you already knew this).

Sadly, no matter how much hype there is about various diets and strategies, the *only* way you can *gain* weight, is if you eat *more* calories than you burn.

And, consequently, the *only* way you can *lose* weight, is if you eat *less* calories than you burn. *It's simple physics.*

One pound of fat is approximately equal to 3,500 calories (half a kilogram equals 3,850 calories). So, to lose one pound (or half a kilogram) of body fat per week, you need a deficit of 3,500-3,850 calories over the seven days, or about 500-550 fewer calories per day.

As a rule of thumb, weight loss is generally 75 to 80 percent diet. Therefore, combining diet with purposeful, physical activity will help you burn more calories.

It is also important that you look after your overall nutrition while you lose weight. Although it is true that a calorie is a calorie no matter the food source, you need to ensure that, at the same time as losing weight, you're still providing your body with the sustenance it needs to be able to function well.

Understanding the role of foods that have fewer calories but are nutritionally dense is essential to your success.

And for any weight loss to be sustainable, its foundations must also be underpinned by good sleep, stress management, and low alcohol intake.

✓ Know your starting point

Being honest about your body measurements can be a confronting exercise. But knowing them is necessary to show your weight right now and to give you a clear picture of your body fat composition.

The best time to measure your body is as you start out on your weight-loss journey so you can see, over time, the positive impact that your healthy eating is having.

First, weigh yourself (correctly)
Knowing your weight provides a simple baseline measure:
- Use the same scales every time (you are only interested in change)
- Get on and off the scales three times to make sure they give a consistent reading
- Weigh at the same time of day and under the same conditions (such as on a hard floor surface)

Then, graph your weight
- Draw a line of your goal weight on a weight graph (this will help to keep you focused)
- Record your weight immediately after you weigh yourself (for accuracy)
- Understand that your weight can show ups and downs which may not be related to fat loss or gain – it could instead be due to how much you are drinking or the weight of undigested food

Next, measure your waist circumference
A tape measure is one of the most useful assessment tools. Measuring your waist circumference is a more accurate predictor of your risk of chronic disease than either your weight by itself or your Body Mass Index, while also giving you a simple measure of your progress.

To accurately measure your waist circumference:
- Stand up straight and breath out
- Position the tape measure halfway between your lowest rib and the top of your hipbone, which should be roughly in line with your belly button
- Place the tape measure directly against your skin so that it is snug but doesn't compress it

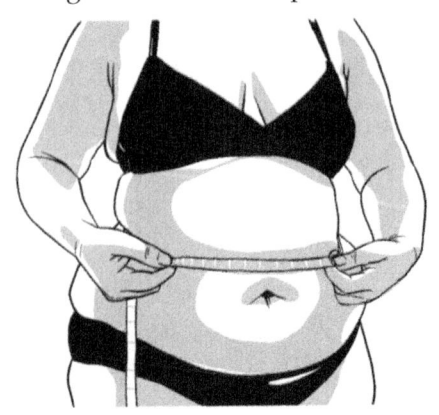

Step 2: Take Control (& Set Yourself Up for Success)

Waist Circumference Health Risk (Women)	
Low Risk	Below 31.5 inches (< 80 centimeters)
Moderate Risk	31.5 to 35 inches (80 to 88 centimeters)
High Risk	35 inches or above (> 88 centimeters)

Now, calculate your Body Mass Index (BMI)

BMI is one way to assess whether your weight is or isn't in the healthy weight range.

To calculate your BMI, either:
1. Measure your weight in pounds and your height in inches.
2. Multiply your weight by 703 and divide it by the square of your height (pounds x 703/inches^2).

or…
1. Measure your weight in kilograms and your height in meters.
2. Divide your weight by the square of your height (kilograms/meters^2).

Body Mass Index	Weight Range
18.5 to 24.9	Normal
25.0 to 30.0	Overweight
30.0 or more	Obese

Next, calculate your waist-to-hip ratio (WHR)

Your health is affected by where you store body fat. WHR measures the ratio of your waist and hip circumference and shows how much fat is stored on your waist, hips, and buttocks. Higher ratios can indicate a higher risk to your health.

WHR is calculated by dividing your waist circumference by your hip circumference.

Fat, Frumpy & Over 50

To calculate your WHR:
1. Measure your waist circumference (as before).
2. Measure your hip circumference, that is, the distance around the largest part of your hips (widest part of your buttocks).
3. Divide your waist by your hip circumference.

Waist-To-Hip Ratio	Health Risk (Women)
0.80 or lower	Low
0.81 to 0.85	Moderate
0.86 or higher	High

Now, measure your skinfold thickness
Measuring your skinfold thickness provides an estimate of your total body fat percentage.

Skinfold calipers are used to measure four skinfolds:
- Biceps (front of middle upper arm)
- Triceps (back of middle upper arm)
- Subscapular (under lowest point of shoulder blade)
- Suprailiac (above upper bone of the hip)

Your skinfold thickness is measured by pinching the skin at these sites and pulling it away from the underlying muscle so only the skin and fat tissue are being held. The measurement is then read by age and sex using the Table of Durnin en Womersly, 1974.)

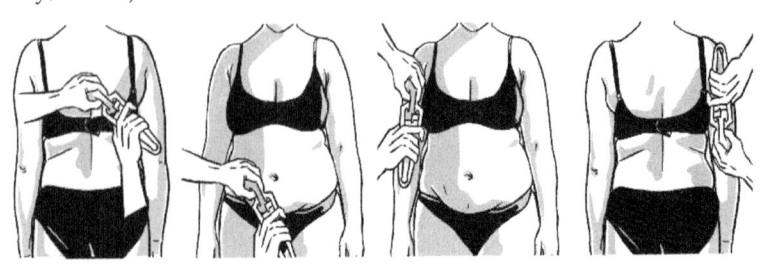

Step 2: Take Control (& Set Yourself Up for Success)

✓ Calculate the calories you need each day

Excess weight can often be caused by unintentional overeating, or rather, by an error in judgement. If you miscalculate your daily calorie intake by a large slice of bread (80 calories), then multiply this by seven days, you will end up with 560 extra calories per week. Repeat this every week over three months and you will consume over 7,000 extra calories which is equivalent to nearly two pounds (one kilogram) of extra body fat. Repeating this for a year is equivalent to eight pounds (about four kilograms) of extra body fat.

Before you set out to lose weight, it's a good idea to know what your calorie intake is now. Track your calories for a typical day or two (a short-term exercise) to give you the baseline information you need to plan what you will eat. You can keep track by hand or use one of the many readily-available free apps or online programs.

The next thing is to calculate how many calories you need to consume each day.

This is a two-step process:
1. Calculate your Basal Metabolic Rate (BMR), that is, how many calories you need just to keep you alive (as if all you're doing is lying on the couch and breathing).
2. Calculate your Total Daily Energy Expenditure (TDEE), that is, how many calories you need when you're up and about and moving around, by multiplying your BMR times your level of physical activity.

The final number you get will give you an estimate of the calorie requirements (TDEE) needed to *maintain* your weight.

To *lose weight* at a sustainable and realistic rate of about one pound (half a kilogram) per week so you *don't lose muscle*, subtract 500 to give you the total calories you will need to consume each day.

Online BMR and TDEE calculators are available (as well as direct calorimetry testing, however this can be expensive). If, instead, you want to understand how it is done, and calculate your basal metabolic rate and recommended daily calorie intake for yourself, here is the formula:

Step 1: Calculate your BMR (for women)

Use the Harris Benedict Formula to calculate the minimum energy your body requires from food to sustain life

BMR = 655.10 + (4.35 x weight in pounds)
+ (4.70 x height in inches) − (4.68 x age in years)

or

BMR = 447.593 + (9.247 x weight in kg)
+ (3.098 x height in cm) − (4.330 x age in years)

Step 2: Use your BMR to calculate your TDEE

Use the Mifflin-St. Jeor formula to multiply your BMR by your level of activity to determine your daily calorie needs

TDEE = BMR x your level of activity (below)

x	x	x	x	x
1.2	**1.375**	**1.55**	**1.725**	**1.9**
Sedentary (little or no exercise)	Light (light exercise 1-3 days a week)	Moderate (moderate exercise 3-5 days a week)	Very active (hard exercise 6-7 days a week)	Extra active (very hard exercise, physical job)

✓ Lose weight, but don't look older

Okay, so to not look frumpy you want to lose those excess pounds. But you also don't want to lose too much fat where you still need it.

Step 2: Take Control (& Set Yourself Up for Success)

Here's what to do:
- Aim for a BMI in the mid to high end of your healthy weight range
- Take your time and aim for one pound (half a kilogram) of weight loss a week to give your skin, especially on your face and stomach, time to adjust
- Eat plenty of protein rich foods (including oily fish)
- Avoid yo-yo dieting at all costs (and its impact on your skin elasticity)
- Eat foods that are good for your gut (leafy greens, whole grains, yogurt, etc.) and have lots of fiber
- Get your aerobic exercise, but don't overdo it – think long walks and slow jogs rather than intense cardio
- Eat plenty of Vitamin C (strawberries, citrus, etc.)
- Treat yourself to 2 to 4 cups a day of green tea (the active ingredient EGCG is a natural antioxidant)
- And, most importantly, *start straight away* – the longer you leave it the greater the loss of skin elasticity

✅ Know your macronutrient requirements

Not all calories in food are created equal. Foods are made up of three macronutrients – carbohydrates, fats, and proteins – and micronutrients – vitamins, minerals and phytochemicals.

Macronutrient	Calories per gram
Protein	4
Carbohydrates	4
Fat	9

Despite your body not recognizing food as 'good' or 'bad' for weight loss (only the calories count), consuming enough nutrient-dense foods and high-quality protein in your diet is essential to give you the 'best bang for your buck'. This is critical for reducing age-related muscle loss, and providing you with optimum energy which will then curb your appetite so you won't feel hungry.

Once you know your TDEE (see page 35), you can calculate your specific macronutrient requirements.

For women over 50, to lose weight consume
25-30% of your calories from protein
45% of your calories from carbohydrates
25-30% of your calories from healthy fats

If consuming 1,600 calories each day, aim for
100-120 grams of protein
180 grams of carbohydrates
45-54 grams of healthy fats

✅ Your week on a plate

Meal planning is instrumental in creating the calorie deficit you require for weight loss, and for giving yourself an advantage going into each week.

Planning your meals in advance:
- Gives you control over your eating habits (you'll always know what's for breakfast, lunch and dinner)
- Increases the likelihood you will stick to your calorie-intake goal, and decreases the chance of making poor food choices
- Helps you avoid mindless eating (a meal plan makes you aware of all your meals and snacks and keeps you accountable to yourself)

Step 2: Take Control (& Set Yourself Up for Success)

- Provides for nutrient-dense meals (based on foods that are high in nutrients but relatively low in calories)
- Reduces decision fatigue about what you will cook and then having to find something last minute
- Takes the stress out of shopping (with a meal plan for the week ahead you know exactly what is on the shopping list while also reducing impulse purchases)
- Helps you avoid getting ravenous (keeping you strong enough to stay on track)

To plan your meals, use either a meal planner tool, or an app such as: *Plan to Eat, Mealtime, MealPrepPro, Make My Plate, Lose It!* or *Eat This Much*.

You can also use a food swap app – which provides nutritional information based on scientific algorithms – to help you compare and make the best food choices.

A guide for spreading your calories across the day (for a 1,600-calorie meal plan)		
Meal	% of daily calories	Approximately
Breakfast	20%	300 calories
Lunch	30%	500 calories
Dinner	40%	600 calories
Snacks	10%	200 calories

✓ Prepare your meals

Meal preparation – 'meal prep' – of some, part or all of your meals in advance will help you to lose weight through calorie and portion control (while also saving you time with batch cooking).

> *If you're struggling to make meal preparation a habit, remind yourself that you're making life easier for your future self.*
> **Heidi Sze, ABC Everyday**

Here's what to do:
- Stock up on all the food containers you will need – including travel coolers for 'on-the-go' meals – to help you portion your food, and keep meals readily available
- Standardize your grocery shopping list (for each meal and each recipe)
- Keep a running list of basic ingredients (healthy staples to always have on hand)
- Keep core ingredients for each recipe 'in stock'
- Make sure you have all the cooking equipment you need ready for use
- Invest in a slow cooker and cook while you are out
- Make a regular time to meal prep, and stick to it – pick a time (preferably the same time) each week when you know you'll be able to get it done
- Try to not shop and meal prep on the same day
- Do as much pre-prep as you can by slicing and cooking ahead of time (chop onions, carrots, celery, etc., keep in sealed containers/bags in measured portions, and then use straight from the freezer)
- Soak grains such as brown rice, oats, quinoa or barley in water overnight to reduce cooking time
- Prepare lunches ahead of time (grain salads can be packed into individual containers with a dressing on the side, eggs boiled, hummus portioned for serving with crackers, etc.)

- Make meal prep sessions an enjoyable experience (maybe listen to some music, or a podcast).

Cook once, eat for days.

✅ Shapeshifters

Be aware of what you're drinking, too.

Wine, beer, cider and spirits are made from natural starch and sugar. This is why alcohol contains so many calories, in fact seven calories per gram (almost the same as fat).

Try to:
- Adjust ingredients in mixed drinks by using more ice or sparkling water and less soda or juice
- Replace high calorie sugars or syrups with fresh herbs such as rosemary, mint or basil to enhance the flavor of your drink

> 'Calories' are the unit of measure used in this book. To convert calories to kilojoules, multiply by 4.184.

✅ Maybe you need extra support from a weight-loss program to get you started

For the majority of women, losing weight is not easy – it takes time, commitment, and hard work, and is full of ups and downs – but it doesn't have to be difficult. It's all about finding an eating plan, and the support, that works for *you*.

One of the biggest struggles can be simply getting started. The next is choosing from the overwhelming number of options telling you what to eat, what not to eat, and when and how to exercise.

If you've decided that you need extra support from a weight-loss program to help you get started or to stay on track – or you're considering ready-made calorie and portion-controlled meals – here are a few (of several) options:

Program only
- WW (Weight Watchers)
- Noom
- Mayo Clinic
- Mighty Health

Meals only
- The Good Kitchen
- Nutrisystem

Program + Meals
- Jenny Craig
- Optavia
- WW (but only limited meals)

✅ More tips for losing weight after 50

Learn to enjoy strength training

As you age, your muscle mass declines. This loss of muscle begins around the age of 50 – with muscle mass decreasing by about 1 to 2% a year, and muscle strength declining at a rate of 1.5 to 5% a year – and can slow your metabolism. This can then lead to weight gain (one pound of muscle burns six calories while one pound of fat burns only four calories).

Strength training can help you lose weight by reducing body fat while maintaining muscle mass and therefore boosting metabolism.

Step 2: Take Control (& Set Yourself Up for Success)

So, add muscle-building strength training exercises to your routine to reduce the impact of age-related muscle loss.

Consider a Mediterranean diet
The Mediterranean diet is touted as the healthiest way of eating and, as it is anti-inflammatory and rich in antioxidants, can be especially beneficial for skin health.

Or look into the 'epigenetics diet'
Epigenetics is the study of how your behaviors and environment can cause changes that affect the way your genes work. Adopting a healthy diet can slow epigenetic age acceleration (crucial for maintaining healthy ageing).

Get enough sleep
You snooze… you lose, and this is a *good* thing. Getting enough quality sleep is an important part of a healthy weight-loss plan to help regulate the hormones that control your appetite and strengthen your willpower.

Not getting enough sleep can inadvertently cause weight gain. And, vice versa, being overweight can affect your sleep.

Hydrate, hydrate, hydrate
Stay hydrated. Drinking plenty of water will help keep your skin hydrated and plumped.

Focus on your skin care
Do everything you can to minimize sun damage. If you're going outside more to walk and exercise, then 'slip, slop, slap, slide': slip on a (collared) shirt, slop on sunscreen, slap on a hat, and slide on sunglasses during the day.

Consider topical applications of products containing hyaluronic acid, peptides, retinol, vitamins A, B3 and C as well as cosmetic treatments involving lasers and fillers as they may help tighten any sagging skin as you lose weight.

Reduce stress and 'feed' your positive

Do what you can to avoid or minimize that 'vicious cycle' between stress, an increase in appetite and weight gain. Whether it's the result of high levels of the stress hormone cortisol, or unhealthy stress-induced behaviors such as unhealthy snacking, or a combination of the two, do what you can to break the cycle.

The bottom line? More stress = more cortisol = higher appetite for junk food = excess body fat.

Step 3: Stay on Track (& Conquer Your Inner Voice)

You've had a reality check about staying overweight and you've set yourself up for success. Now it's about giving yourself every chance of *finally* succeeding.

No matter how prepared you are, in the early days, food cravings can still occur and will try to knock you off track, at least until you've locked in your new routines and habits, and made some tangible progress with losing weight (which in itself will motivate you to stay the course).

So, right now, you'll need a bucketload of strategies to make sure you crush those cravings and keep yourself on track.

Step 3 supports you to:
- *Prevent* cravings taking hold of you in the first place, and
- Crush your cravings *in-the-moment* to quickly get you out of 'craving mode', and back on track

Step 3: Stay on Track (& Conquer Your Inner Voice)

Part 1: <u>Prevent</u> food cravings <u>before</u> they take hold of you

The vast majority of us experience cravings… that intense urge to consume a particular, usually unhealthy, food, regardless of how hungry or full we are. You are not alone!

The best approach is to prevent them *before* they get you in their sight. Without a doubt, the easiest craving to resist is the one that never grabs you in the first place.

So, right now, to avoid any cravings grabbing hold of you, take some time to get your *preventative* strategies in place.

✅ First of all, face up to your future self

I imagine you have felt unique in experiencing the excitement over and over again of getting ready to finally succeed and lose weight 'this time' (the whole idea of succeeding is wildly exciting). The dreams of how you will look and feel after you have lost that weight are captivating.

But then, time and time again, reality kicks in and you realize you actually have to commit to doing something different to succeed, something that requires effort and giving up on your familiar, comforting but unhealthy food choices and habits.

And, as it gets harder to do what you need to do to lose weight *right now*, you surrender (again) to the present, and give in to eating that [fill in the gap] sitting right there in front of you.

But then, almost without pause, the next wave of excitement begins to stir, that rekindling of hope to start again (next Monday?) because, you know 'without a doubt', *you will succeed next time.*

In the moment that you decide to eat that [fill in the gap], you are again putting more value in immediate gratification and less in your potential future rewards (and all for about three minutes of bliss!). What you are doing is called 'delay discounting', where you think (and believe) you can, and will, 'do it later'.

To win this battle against your present self, you are going to have to *face up to your future self*.

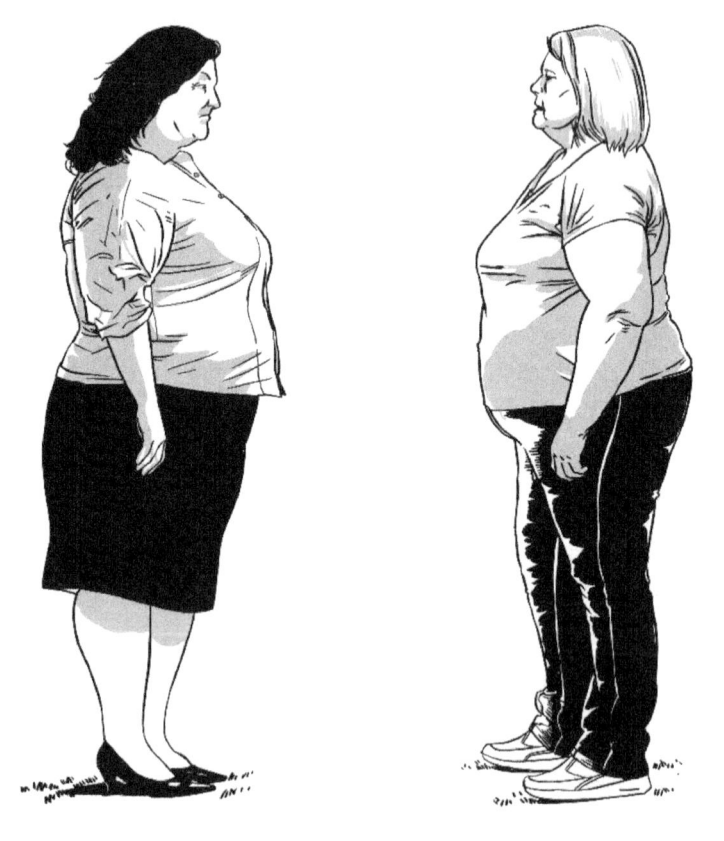

Meeting your future self... AND NOT IMPRESSED!

Step 3: Stay on Track (& Conquer Your Inner Voice)

Start by taking a journey to your future self
Ask yourself, "What does my future self look like 10 years from now?".

Imagine if, between now and then, you *made positive choices and maintained a healthy weight*. Picture how your life has changed from what it is like today.

Next, imagine if instead, throughout those 10 years, you have *continued with your unhealthy eating as you are doing now and have changed nothing*. How do you look? And, more importantly, how do you feel?

To connect with your future self, try this exercise:
1. Get into a comfortable position, put your hands on your lap, close your eyes and take a couple of deep breaths.
2. Picture the pages of a calendar scrolling ahead 10 years, one month after the other.
3. Assume that all of those years have been *massively successful* and you are a healthy weight.
4. Answer the following questions (just the first thoughts that come to mind):
    - Where am I? What is happening around me?
    - How would I describe myself? What do I look like, act like, dress like?
    - Who am I with? What are my relationships like? Intimate? Family? Friends?
    - How am I feeling? Am I happy?
5. Stay in the future for a while, soak it up and sit with your answers before picturing the calendar flipping back to the present day, then slowly open your eyes.
6. Reflect on how you saw your future self… on all that was positive and all that felt good.
7. Hang on to that feeling of an amazing future, keep it in your conscious mind and *treat it as if it is now*.

Next, write letters from your future self

This can be such a deep, reflective and joyous process and can bring about a powerful mindset shift. Write to yourself with love. Write for whatever time periods you feel will motivate you the most.

Dear [your name],

Picture it. Today is the 1st [month] [year], *just over one year from the day I decided to live the life that I am capable of living,* it is a [day of the week] and it's the first day of [season].

My weight now is [your weight] and I am fitter today than I have been in years. I continue to stick to all my wellbeing goals. My social life is full and fun. I am keeping my options open for having an intimate relationship again.

Life is good. I am so happy and excited with how I am living it. I feel fabulous. I am grateful for the richness of my life.

Lots of love
[your name] xx

Dear [your name],

Picture it. The year is [year]. Today is the 1st [month] [year*]*, *10 years from the day I decided to live the life that I am capable of living,* it is a [day of the week] and it's sunny.

My weight has been stable at [your weight] for many years now. I am fit, active and I feel fabulous. I continue to stick to all my wellbeing goals. I have an active social life, and have been in a loving relationship for over eight years.

Life is good. I am so happy and excited now and for what's to come. I am grateful for the richness of my life.

Lots of love
[your name] xx

Step 3: Stay on Track (& Conquer Your Inner Voice)

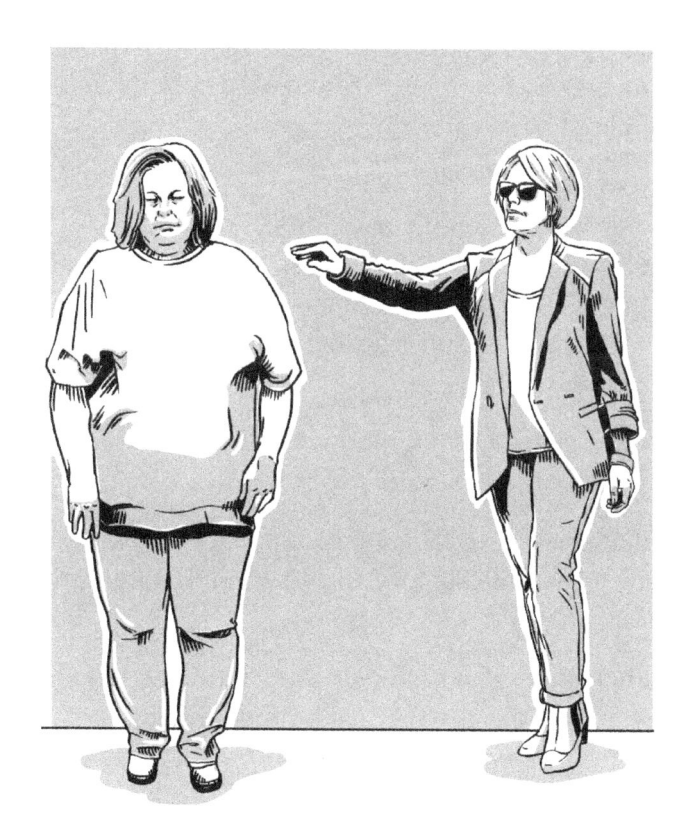

Let your future self reach out to you

✓ Win over your (lack of) willpower

Jennifer, a smart, accomplished woman, who understands the health risks of being overweight, decides to tackle her excess weight and to jump start her weight loss with intermittent fasting (she had read about the success of the 16:8 diet). She works out a meal plan and stocks up her pantry. She feels excited about what's ahead and is ready to go. And for a couple of weeks, she sticks to her plan.

And then what happens? It is 7pm, she is just home from

work, no dinner planned, it's outside her 'fasting window', she is tired, stressed, overwhelmed and ready for bed… and well, you know the rest.

Does she:
1. Decide not to eat until breakfast?
2. Cook a healthy meal anyway and eat it outside her fasting window? *or* (correct answer)
3. Opt for her tried-and-true Mexican takeaway (with all the add-ons, of course)?

After a few weeks her willpower has crumpled, and her weight-loss goals are back on the 'to do' list.

Is Jennifer weak and completely lacking self-control? Or is she, instead, just putting too much faith in the strength of her willpower.

Although some women have strong willpower, the majority of us don't. And this is where *habit* comes into play.

As it happened, Jennifer set her goals when she was enthusiastic and in a motivated state of mind. And now, when she is tired, stressed and overwhelmed, she is relying solely on her willpower when, most likely, she isn't still feeling that same high she felt when she first committed to her goals.

If, instead, she had established different habits and developed new behaviors (including preparing in advance to have a healthy meal available), she would have needed to make much less of a conscious effort when she was tired and overwhelmed, as her new habit and behaviors would already be well on the way to becoming automatic.

That's because her brain would have set about establishing 'shortcuts' that supported these new habits and it wouldn't have required so much conscious thought (our brain always wants to be efficient and repeat the same behaviors over and over). When Jennifer relied only on willpower, the outcome was always going to depend on her state-of-mind *at that time*.

Habits are behaviors – both wanted and unwanted – that have become increasingly automatic because you have consistently engaged in them in the same situation over a period of time.

But your unwanted habits can be outsmarted.

To do this you will need to:
- *Break into* your consciousness and *remake* them (to change your brain's 'shortcut')
- Find your *activation energy* to overcome resistance to doing something you are currently doing without conscious thought to doing something new

The approach to shattering your current unwanted habits works best when you:
- Focus on one thing at a time
- Are realistic about the scale of change, and
- Allow enough time for the new behavior to become a habit

Here's how to outsmart your unwanted habits

Step 1: Take time to become *aware* of the behavior you want to change and decide on the new habit that will replace it.

Step 2: *Identify* the cue, trigger, sequence or circumstance that leads to your unwanted behavior (this could be location, time, stress, boredom, anxiety, a smell, sound or sight, other people, or something that has just happened).

Step 3: *Interrupt* your behavior pattern *immediately* in the instant that it happens.
- Stop right away then delay by telling yourself you are not giving in to it right now

- Do something different that satisfies your trigger but also supports your goals
- Stay strong (remind yourself that it's harder at the start to overcome resistance, but it will get easier)

Step 4: *Check in* with yourself after 10 to 15 minutes and decide if you still have the urge or if it has been satisfied. If the urge is still there, try something different.

Step 5: Stick with it and r*epeat, repeat, repeat* (something you only do once is not a new habit).

Outsmart Your Bad Habits Template
Step 1: Reflect on the current behavior that you want to change   The habit of having a glass or two of wine every night to relax when I get home from work.
Step 2: Identify the cue, trigger or circumstance that leads to your unwanted behavior   When I get home, I'm feeling stressed and having a glass of wine (almost on auto-pilot) has become the 'thing I do' to help me feel better.
Step 3: Interrupt your behavior pattern   I decide to stop immediately and instead do a short, guided meditation.
Step 4: Check in with yourself after 15 minutes   After 15 minutes, I'm still feeling the urge to have a glass of wine (although it is much less), so straight away I head outside and look at the night sky.
Step 5: Stick with it   Every night for two weeks I have been doing a short meditation when I get home and it is becoming part of my new nightly routine (and is an effective stress reliever).

Step 3: Stay on Track (& Conquer Your Inner Voice)

Practice makes perfect
As well as the unwanted habits you're already working on, setting yourself some 'micro challenges' with simple, everyday tasks will help to strengthen your habit-forming 'muscle'. Getting past any feelings of discomfort will keep reinforcing, in your mind, the effort required to outsmart the habits you want to change.

For instance:
- Get out of bed immediately when you wake up (if you don't already)
- Turn the water to cold for the last 10 seconds of your shower
- Stand up on the bus even if there is a seat available

> *We are what we repeatedly do.*
> *Excellence, therefore, is not an act but a habit.*
> *Aristotle*

✓ Reframe your self-talk

Stay positive and reflect on your accomplishments. Think about your new healthy habits as things you *get* to do rather than things you *have* to do.

Instead of thinking "I can't", ask yourself "Has anyone?" or "Have I ever?" By finding just one example that breaks your belief, you show yourself that the belief is untrue.

> *Lose weight.*
> *Gain confidence.*
> *Not vice versa.*

✓ Get to know your hunger

Recognize whether you are hungry (a physiological 'below-the-neck' need) or if you just have a craving to eat something... anything (an emotional 'above-the-neck' need).

1. Stop for a moment, think about what you're actually feeling and recognize your level of hunger (using the scale below).
2. If you're not actually hungry (Level 6 to 10), see it for what it is and get busy doing something else instead.

Hunger Level Scale	
Hungry	**Not Hungry**
Level 1 Starving, hunger pangs, shaky, light headed	**Level 6** Satisfied
Level 2 Slight stomach pain, hard to concentrate, lack of energy	**Level 7** Feel food in stomach
Level 3 Start of physical signs of hunger, stomach growling	**Level 8** Stomach sticks out
Level 4 Could eat if it were suggested	**Level 9** Bloated, clothes feel tight, sleepy and drained
Level 5 Neutral	**Level 10** Stomach uncomfortable, no energy, physically sick

Do the apple test. Ask yourself would you still want this snack if it were only an apple or raw carrots? If the answer is yes, then it's likely to be physical hunger. If the answer is no, then you're probably experiencing emotional hunger.

✅ Maybe you're only thirsty?

Sometimes when you're stalking the fridge it might be water that you actually need. Dehydration can be surprisingly easily confused with hunger and cravings.

Have a drink of water, then reassess after 15 minutes whether you are actually hungry (and always carry a water bottle with you).

✅ Bundle temptation

One of the best ways to build a new habit is with 'temptation bundling' or 'habit stacking'.

This involves combining a pleasurable, healthy, indulgent behavior that you have already established (a 'want') with a task that you are struggling to start or stick with that provides longer term rewards (a 'need').

The temptation bundling + habit stacking formula is:
1. After [my current habit], I will [the new habit I need to establish].
2. After [the new habit I need to establish], I will [the indulgence I want].

For example, if you want to listen to your favorite podcast, but you need to do meal prep:
1. After I take my dog for a walk on Sunday, I will start my meal prep for the week ahead (a 'need' behavior).
2. After I start my meal prep, I will listen to my favorite podcast (the indulgence I want).

You can also link micro habits within your existing routine. Take any new behavior, scale it back into bite-sized chunks that take you less than 30 seconds to do and require little effort, then link them in with something you already do.

For instance, it could be something as simple as having a drink of water when you wake up instead of going straight for a cup of coffee in the morning.

✓ Establish non-negotiable rules

Iron-clad rules are good for busting emotional eating. Just like Finnish people's special kind of resilience, Sisu, which focuses on having grit and perseverance in the face of challenges, establish your own rules. Then dig deep and stick to them.

Maybe...
- "I will walk for 30 minutes every day."
- "I will not eat in front of the TV."
- "I will not sit in my car and eat."
- "I will not eat later than 6.00pm."

> **YOUR MESSAGE IS SIMPLE:**
> *If you're overweight,* **DON'T EAT JUNK FOOD.**
> *If you're overweight, and you do eat junk food,* **STOP.**
> *If you don't stop eating junk food,* **CHANGE.**

✓ Use pain to propel you forward instead of allowing it to hold you back

Be aware that you are always on a *pain versus pleasure* pendulum, where decisions you make are to either avoid pain or to gain pleasure. This awareness will give you the power to make choices.

To help you truly choose the actions that you want to take in relation to being overweight, ask yourself, "What is the pain

Step 3: Stay on Track (& Conquer Your Inner Voice)

of *not* losing weight? Of *not* taking action?" It is only when you acknowledge just how much pain is associated with your inaction (of staying overweight), and that the pain is intolerable, that you can move forward. It's when you reach that point that you are able to decide, "I've had enough!"

Complete the following statement:
"If I don't take action right now, I will experience [fill in your pain]".

It could be…
- "I will be stuck in a tedious cycle of endlessly restarting a diet nearly every Monday."
- "I will stay overweight and continue to be an 'invisible' middle-aged woman."
- "I will risk becoming unwell and no longer have the option of living the life that I want."

And then, be strong! You will have to constantly choose between instant gratification – fun and easy pleasure, *right now* – or, your *future* pleasure. Remind yourself that choosing instant gratification now is also about making a choice for future pain.

Sometimes, life is like needing to go to the toilet in the middle of the night… you really don't want to get up and do it, but you feel so much better when you have.
Gretel Killeen

✓ Know your end date

To keep you motivated, have a realistic plan, not only for when you start on your weight-loss journey, but also for when you expect to cross the finish line.

✅ Write your own 'before' and 'after' story

If you want to live differently and feel more successful in your life, first you must begin to show up as that version of yourself. You have to play the role.

So, get inspired by writing your own weight-loss success story by telling it as though you have already reached your goal.

If you're wondering how to write it, look at other women's real-life before and after stories and use them as a guide (check out the WW website).

✅ Always remind yourself why you are doing this

To keep your focus on your future benefit, keep your goals front of mind. Regularly think about them so they can have a greater effect on your consciousness.

Keep reminding your *current self* that your *future self* will be so thankful for it.

✅ Aim high and make a declaration

You could declare that the next 12 months is going to be your 'Year of Health'.

✅ Take on a challenge

A few ideas…
- Challenge yourself at 57 to fit into the jeans you wore when you were 20 (and rock your new look)
- Enter a 30-day fitness challenge to do at least 10,000 steps every day

- Print a map, draw a 5-mile (8-kilometer) circle from your home, and aim to walk every street (and mark them off as you go)
- Or perhaps you could join 'parkrun', an international ultra-inclusive movement where everyone is welcome and you set the pace. Turn up each Saturday and walk, jog or run. That's it. At your own speed. Totally free. (The aim of parkrun is to create a healthier, happier planet for everyone.)

A 60-minute 5km (3.1 mile) walk is just as far as a 15-minute 5km run.

✓ Limit your time by setting a deadline

Give yourself the gift of desperation. Lock in a non-negotiable deadline, either one that fills you with dread or one that excites you, so that you will *have* to get this (weight loss) done.

If you don't have any actual deadlines right now (apart from your future health), come up with one. Perhaps,

"It's 12 weeks to Christmas, and I can't wait to see the look on the faces of my family when I walk in all fit and fabulous."

✓ Create a little competition

Think about entering into a contract with a friend, where you compete against each other to stick to your weight-loss plan. To get the best from yourself compete against someone who is even more motivated than you. Agree on a prize that is significant enough to keep you both on track. And make it real so that you actually payout if you lose – although, of course, the goal is for both of you to win!

✓ Make it easier to avoid temptation

Don't make things harder for yourself, make them easier. Aim to eliminate or avoid temptation instead of trying to ignore or block it out. Keep yourself away from willpower challenges.

For instance, don't go to a bakery for a coffee when you're trying to avoid the cheesecake.

✓ Plan for a future event

Stay focused on an event where you know you'll want to look your absolute best. Maybe have the ticket or invitation nearby to keep that feeling tangible.

✓ Look good in front of an ex

Eek!!! You've bumped into one of your exes! Do you want to show them how great you are (and feel) or will you be heading for the door, hoping you haven't been seen?

If being healthy, confident and super-stylish is how you want to be when you see an ex, don't risk not doing what you need to do while you still have time.

Create scenarios in your mind where you meet one of your exes and you're looking fabulous. Visualize it, feel it, and keep it front of mind (so there's no more heading for the door).

> *We met in a carpark… and I remember thinking that I'd want to do my hair nicely if I was to bump into him again.*
> **Lucy Durack**

Step 3: Stay on Track (& Conquer Your Inner Voice)

✅ Do it for sweet revenge

"Dumped Wife Gets Best Revenge on Her Ex-Husband"

This is what Dianne Laurence had to say:
"After 26 years together, my husband left me for the younger women. I decided within weeks of the initial shock and trauma what my revenge was going to be, I was going to be fabulous and look fabulous.

The best and only revenge to have when you get hit with a curveball that knocks you back on your butt is to get back and be fabulous. The best revenge for being dumped by a partner or when life dumps on you is to always be your fabulous best and the world of wondrous opportunities will open."
(dumpedwifesrevenge.com)

✅ Make a commitment contract with yourself

A 'Self-Contract' is a tool that can help you truly commit to your goal of being a healthy weight.

Although the idea is to focus on making positive changes in your life, you can sometimes make your contract more effective by creating a penalty if you don't stick to your goal. (Maybe having to cancel something you are reeaallly looking forward to?)

✅ Make sure you have something to look forward to every day

Anticipation is a powerful feeling. It can be inspiring and energizing. Think about the things that give you joy, and make them part of your (every) day.

Before you go to bed, remind yourself what will get you out of bed in the morning, ready to seize the day? Maybe the jumbo coffee you reward yourself with each morning?

✅ Do it with a like-minded buddy

Find someone to come along with you because when you're a team of only one, no one notices if you go off track.

✅ Surround yourself with 'healthy' people making positive decisions

Be aware of 'mirroring' an overweight friend or sibling. The health decisions and behaviors they exhibit can unconsciously influence the choices you make.

✅ Use a 'motivation motivator'

There are various tools available to help keep you motivated. They work by getting your mind to pay attention to the feedback they provide.

Fitness trackers (wearable activity trackers) and fitness apps motivate you to move more. They provide constant feedback and keep you accountable (to yourself). Once your mind begins paying attention to the device around your wrist or on your phone, building habits such as walking more or making healthier food choices become easier.

Body composition scales measure how much of your weight is body fat, fat free mass – including muscle – and water, in addition to your total weight.

The mPort 3D body scanner (known as 'mPod') uses infrared sensors to map and provide 3D images of your body and includes comparison views. Graphs of your body composition (including body fat estimates) are also included. This enables you to visualize and measure changes in your body, and track your progress.

Alternatively, Bodymapp, utilizing the mPort app on your phone, uses a depth sensor to map the external contours of your body and transform it into a 3D bodymesh that matches your true body shape (the advantage of this body scan is that you can do it at home.)

✓ Join a local online community of supportive women (or create one)

Talk to like-minded women to seek motivation and to share your story (and all while showing kindness and encouragement to others).

You could set up a private Facebook group to help you stay accountable to a small, trusted cohort.

✓ Enlist a mentor

Think about someone in your life who inspires you. Talk to them. Find out about their strengths (and weaknesses). Ask them to be your mentor.

✓ Ask for feedback

Seek support from a close, trusted friend. Ask them how they see your behaviors as well as your strengths and weaknesses.

Other people can see patterns of behavior where you haven't supported yourself and can bring these blind spots into your awareness.

✅ Join a campaign

Wellbeing *can* exist on social media in a way that isn't potentially damaging. Have you heard of the 'This Girl Can' campaign? It aims to inspire women to be more physically active and is a "sassy celebration of active women everywhere".

✅ Make it public

To keep yourself accountable, go public. Maybe start your own Instagram page? Or, attend an in-person weight-loss program such as WW (Weight Watchers).

✅ Plan ahead to make the most of every day

What you consistently do on a daily basis will determine your weight-loss success.

As tempting as it is to tell yourself you'll just "get around" to the things you need to do such as meal planning, meal prep and getting enough exercise, the reality is that when you get busy these are the first tasks to get lost in the shuffle.

Planning your day ahead, every day, is key to taking control. Prioritizing the tasks that support your weight loss is ultimately essential to your success.

And, do your planning the night before to give yourself a heads up on what tomorrow will look like. You will be mentally prepared the moment you wake up.

> *How we spend our days is, of course, how we spend our lives.*
> **Annie Dillard**

✓ Prioritize your sleep (you don't stand a chance if you're tired!)

You will have an even tougher time losing weight if you are sleep deprived. You tend to crave foods that are high in calories and carbohydrates if you are tired, and your motivation crumbles.

- Plan for regular sleep and aim for the same time to bed and getting up (allowing at least seven hours of sleep each night)
- Finish eating three hours before your bedtime
- And if you can, be an 'early-to-bed' person (you are more likely to consume extra calories if you go to bed late)

✓ Move it

Exercise offers significant benefits for women over 50.

Although it can help you to lose weight, exercise is even more important for your overall health and wellbeing as it contributes to lowering your risk of developing chronic illnesses such as heart disease, diabetes and osteoporosis (certain types of exercise, particularly weight-bearing, can help improve your bone health). You can also restore lost muscle (even well into your 90s). But probably the most significant benefit is that it can make you feel great about yourself.

If you were physically active before 50, that's great. But if you didn't exercise regularly, it's not too late to start.

The amount of exercise recommended for women over the age of 50 is the same as the amount recommended for women of all ages. Aim for at least 150 minutes of moderate aerobic exercise or 75 minutes of vigorous exercise, each week. That works out to 30 minutes of moderate exercise or 15 minutes of vigorous exercise five days a week.

10 Ways to Burn 100 Calories	
Walking	22 minutes (moderate pace)
Yoga	20 minutes (moderate intensity)
Ironing	34 minutes
Gardening	25 minutes
Climbing stairs	10 minutes
Bike riding	13 minutes (light cycling)
Swimming	15 minutes (moderate intensity)
Tennis	11 minutes (game of singles)
Dancing	20 minutes
Zumba	9 minutes

The four main types of exercise for women over 50 are:
1. Aerobic/cardiovascular (endurance exercises), that you maintain for at least 10 minutes, such as walking, running, cycling or swimming.
2. Strength training (resistance and lifting weights) such as Pilates or using resistance bands.
3. Stretching, to improve and maintain flexibility, such as yoga.
4. Balance, to maintain and improve coordination and to build core strength and body alignment. A simple exercise can be standing on one leg. If you can reach 10 seconds with your eyes closed, you're doing well – the trick is to embrace the wobble. (Balance starts to decline somewhere between 40 to 50 years of age – practising the one leg stance is an opportunity to recalibrate your brain.)

Step 3: Stay on Track (& Conquer Your Inner Voice)

✅ Align with an inspirational celebrity (of a similar age)

Follow them on Instagram, Facebook – but keep it positive and real – it's likely they have a lot more support than you.

✅ Practice first aid for your mind, body and soul

Three things you can practice every day to improve your emotional wellbeing and, as a result, your relationship with food, include:

1. Mindfulness

Mindfulness is about purposely paying attention to what you are doing in the moment.

Mindful eating is eating with awareness and having a better relationship with food.

Mindfulness techniques can help you understand what's behind your urge to eat (when you're not actually hungry), so you can create new, healthier eating habits.

Mindful Eating Awareness
- Engage as many of your senses as possible – notice colors, sounds, textures, smells, and tastes (for example, as you drink a cup of coffee it could be the rising steam, the feel of the cup, the strong aroma, or its warmth and taste on your tongue)
- Pay attention to the effects particular foods have on your feelings and body

Mindful Eating Techniques
- Sit down at an actual table – avoid eating standing up or on the go

- Turn off your phone, TV, computer, etc. – eating while distracted can drown out your 'stop eating' messages
- Pause briefly to observe your food before you start to eat
- Take a moment to smell and taste your food
- Eat more slowly to allow your body to respond to cues (eating faster results in eating more – it takes approximately 20 minutes from the time you start eating for your brain to send out signals of fullness)
- Chew thoroughly (at least 20 chews per bite)
- Put your knife and fork down between each mouthful
- Observe the Japanese tradition of hara hachi bu (eating until you're 80% full and then stopping) to allow your body a chance to catch up so you don't overeat
- Leave one or two mouthfuls (simple but effective)
- Enjoy meals with other people when you can
- Create and keep to a mealtime routine by eating at roughly the same time each day.

2. Gratitude

Gratitude is the simple process of adopting an 'abundance mindset', remembering that your life is good and that you have enough, while also bringing more of what you want into your life (including sticking to your goal of being a healthy weight).

> *If you go to bed with gratitude,*
> *you wake up with inspiration.*
> **Dr John Demartini**

Step 3: Stay on Track (& Conquer Your Inner Voice)

Aim to think of one or two things you're grateful for during the day and again before you go to bed. Always add the two most powerful words, "Thank you".

3. Positive affirmations

Affirmations are positive statements that can help you to challenge and overcome self-sabotaging and negative thoughts.

Create affirmations that excite you, such as:
- "I do this for myself and all the people I love."
- "I create my future with the decisions I make now."

As you repeat each affirmation, visualize yourself truly living and embracing the words you are saying.

The more emotion and enthusiasm you put into embodying each one, the more you will get out of them.

✅ Monitor your progress by keeping tangible measurements of yourself

Measurements don't lie. Whether your goal is about losing weight or being healthy (or both), having tangible, visual measurements that change over time can mark your progress and keep you on track.

Aim to…
- Begin today, and then weigh yourself consistently, preferably once a week (see Step 2)
- Log it in an app or on your weight-loss tracker (failure to record your progress can make any changes feel hit-or-miss and not have the same impact)
- Monitor your measurements to keep giving yourself a 'reality check' (and the opportunity to adjust what you're doing if you need to)
- Feel excited by what you have achieved

✅ Have a 12-week check in

12 weeks on… how are you going? Sometimes you can get caught up only in what's going on right now and lose some perspective. It's motivating to be able to step away from your week-to-week measurements and take time to look at your overall weight-loss trend.

✅ Take progress photos of yourself

Create a visual reminder of your transformation. Capture the 'before' you as you start this journey and the 'during' you along the way.

- Take your photo – front-on, side-on, and back-on – in front of a calendar each week, wearing the same clothes and standing in the same position
- Create an album where you can see your progress photos lined up side by side

✅ Create a body transformation video diary

At your six-month mark, compile a 30-second time-lapse video of your weekly progress photos to record your striking transformation. And add your favorite, motivating music track to play along with it.

✅ Make a talking, animated avatar of yourself

Create a computer-generated avatar of yourself with look-alike physical characteristics (hair color, skin color, weight) and eating healthy food or exercising.

Watching 'yourself' can spur on healthier behaviors.

Step 3: Stay on Track (& Conquer Your Inner Voice)

✅ Use your daily food tracker/journal

Keep yourself accountable to an observant yet non-judgmental party (you!)
- Write down everything you eat or use a food tracker app (it's surprising how quickly calories add up)
- Record as you go (for accuracy)
- Make sure you record the correct amounts or portions of each food

✅ Always know how much you're eating

Even if you are using measuring cups and spoons, this still requires some eyeballing and minor differences can add up.

Using a food scale to weigh your food ensures you always know exactly how much you are eating.

✅ Control your portion size

Start with less on your plate.
- When dishing up your meal, serve your portion first, then put any remaining food straight into the fridge or freezer so you don't mindlessly pick at it
- Use smaller plates and bowls (if you eat from a large plate, you are likely to consume as much as 40% more food)
- Measure your meals with a 'Portion Control' tool (amazon.com)

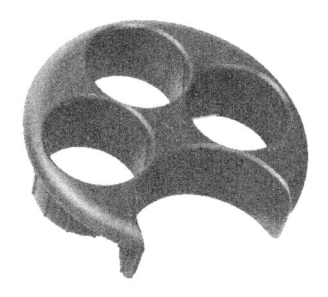

73

> *You better cut the pizza into four pieces because I'm not hungry enough to eat six.*
> **Yogi Berra**

✅ Risk assess yourself

Know your weak times. Maybe 4pm is when a sweet tooth craving hits so be prepared to either distract yourself or have a healthy food option on hand (such as air-popped popcorn).

And don't ever let your blood sugar drop too far as this will only increase the risk of cravings kicking in, especially for sweet foods.

✅ Add flavor, not calories

'Bland' food is your mortal enemy, especially now that you are focused on actually tasting what you're eating (rather than mindlessly gobbling it up).

Boost flavor with fresh herbs, nutmeg, ginger, cinnamon, lemon juice, vinegar, tamari, miso, etc.

✅ Reduce 'decision fatigue'

If you need a break from having to decide what your next meal is going to be, eat the same healthy breakfast, lunch and dinner day after day for a week. Also, have on hand a 'recipe bible' of simple recipes you have tried and tested (including one or two five-minute meals).

If you're unable to cook a meal, and you don't have a pre-prepared meal on hand, just 'assemble' one – simply grab a healthy protein, a healthy fat and a healthy carbohydrate.

Step 3: Stay on Track (& Conquer Your Inner Voice)

'Decision-Fatigue' Cheat Sheet	
Healthy Protein	
Lean beef	Tuna
Chicken breast	Egg whites
White fish	Non-fat Greek yogurt
Healthy Carb	
Wholegrain bread	Peas (legumes)
Oats	Berries
Quinoa	Bananas
Sweet potatoes	Oranges
Healthy Fat	
Avocado	Almonds
Feta	Walnuts
Peanut butter	
Healthy Protein + Healthy Fat	
Salmon	Whole eggs
Tofu	
Healthy Protein + Healthy Carb	
Kidney beans	Soy beans
Chickpeas	Navy beans
Lentils	Fruit & yogurt
Black beans	Eggs on toast

Something else to consider are meal delivery kits. This could help reduce your decision fatigue while also making meal preparation easier, more convenient, and all while channeling your inner chef.

Food is delivered with pre-portioned ingredients and step-by-step instructions for meals that are balanced in terms of macronutrients. Meal kits that are lower in total calories are also available. Another bonus can be the variety of meals on offer from week to week.

✓ Don't eat too late

Technically, the time of day you eat doesn't affect how your body processes food. Eating at night won't make you fat if your overall food intake matches your daily calorie needs. The total amount of calories you take in, and how much you exercise during the day, is what affects your weight.

The problem is that late-night eating patterns – including overeating and choosing high-calorie foods as snacks – can result in the consumption of extra calories and subsequent weight gain.

Even when you eat late meals rather than snacks, you may be very hungry because lunch was such a long time ago, and so you naturally opt for larger portion sizes.

There's also the risk that eating too close to bedtime can actually harm your sleep (which can then impact your weight), especially if you're consuming a large amount of food. When you eat late at night, the muscles that digest and metabolize your food have to keep working when they should be resting. This can delay your ability to fall asleep and prevent you from getting into the deep, restful stage of sleep you need.

So, as a general rule of thumb, wait about three hours between your last meal and bedtime.

If you are still up late – and you ate your dinner earlier – going for an evening walk to fill in the time before bed will take you away from sitting at the table and the temptation to keep picking, picking, picking.

✓ Slow down at meal time

Do anything, basically, that slows down the process of eating:

Step 3: Stay on Track (& Conquer Your Inner Voice)

- Put your cutlery down between each mouthful
- Cut food into smaller pieces
- Have a glass of water with your meal

✓ Have a backup plan when eating away from home

Don't treat eating out as a mini-holiday where you 'go for it'.
- Read the restaurant menu before you arrive so you're mentally prepared and don't have to make any snap decisions
- Order your meal before everyone else to avoid being influenced by their choices
- When it's time for dessert, have a coffee instead, go to the bathroom, sit on your hands or just tell the waiter, "Not for me, thanks."
- When you're travelling, plan ahead, take healthy snacks and try to stick to the same eating schedule you have at home

✓ You can't eat what you don't have

Triple check that there aren't any unhealthy foods within reach in your refrigerator or cupboards that will keep calling out to you "eat me, eat me". Instead, if you still want them, give them to someone else to ration out to you (two Oreos a night could stop you eating the whole packet on auto pilot). And if you have to share your household, keep other people's snacks out of sight (and out of *your* mind).

But don't keep your cupboards bare. If there is no healthy food in the house you will be much more likely to give in and buy junk food or order takeaway. Remember, hunger is not your friend.

Forget the old belief that if you're feeling hungry, you are somehow being a good dieter… it's not true.

It can also help to clean and unclutter your kitchen – messy kitchens can 'uninspire' you and be associated with less healthy eating habits.

✓ Maintain your frightened determination

Keep focusing on what you stand to 'lose'. Create panic! Create fear! Be scared! Remind yourself of the consequences of inaction and why it is so important to overcome it.

Focus on your fear of lost time, and of what you stand to lose (if you don't lose weight). Think about your disappointment; and the hassle of having to start over and over again.

Slap yourself around (metaphorically) and confront yourself when you say "I'll just start again on Monday" (and see it for the cop-out that it is).

✓ Get to know what body fat looks like

Two pounds (about one kilogram) of muscle and two pounds of fat will both weigh two pounds. The difference is in total volume. Two pounds of muscle is about as big as a baseball whereas two pounds of fat is *three times* the size.

✓ Confront yourself with knowing what you're actually doing to your body

Keep reading the facts about health issues related to being overweight – heart disease, high blood pressure, type 2 diabetes, cancer, etc. – and the risks you are taking if you don't change.

Step 3: Stay on Track (& Conquer Your Inner Voice)

Print them out and stick them on your fridge door so they are right there in front of you.

✅ Always think of your weight in pounds – it's easier to put on weight in kilos!

When you are 85 kilograms you don't feel nearly as overweight as you do when you are 187 pounds!

✅ Create your bucket list

Making a bucket list is really about deciding to live life to the full with *all* the days you have left.

Don't wait for that 'perfect time' to tick 'feeling fabulous' off your list.

Write it down or use one of several apps or communities.

'Bucket List' Communities
- Bucketlist.org, Bucketlist.net

'Bucket List' Apps
- BuckitDream, iWish

✅ Have some fun

Join a dance class – a virtual one in your own home (if you want a completely judgement-free zone) – or maybe a class in your local community (giving yourself an opportunity to be sociable, accountable and to enjoy yourself while still taking on a physical challenge). Zumba sounds like fun!

Maybe uncover the delights of learning to make mouthwatering meals in a social cooking class. You could find out about all those best-kept cooking tips and tricks under the guidance of chefs and other passionate foodies. Bon appétit!

✅ Imagine yourself at your own funeral

Confronting your own mortality can have a profound impact on creating a sense of urgency and clarity about your current life, particularly your health and wellbeing.

Imagine looking on at your own funeral after passing away in your 50s. What have you left behind? What regrets do you have? Are you sorry for the actions you took (or didn't take) about your health along the way? Then choose to take action now and regret nothing.

✅ Try on your summer clothes

It's easy to hide your weight under layers of frumpy clothes, but you know it's there.

Trying on your swimsuit every week can give you some added motivation to stay on track.

✅ Surround yourself with words and images that motivate you

Incorporate exhilarating messages into the things you see and use every day.

1. **Display them**
    - Design and print a poster of your 'why' and keep it front and center – reminding yourself of your *purpose* everyday can help to keep you excited when you're dealing with the not-so-fun aspects of losing weight
    - Create a coffee mug with a motivational message on it or maybe a fridge magnet or new screensaver

Step 3: Stay on Track (& Conquer Your Inner Voice)

- Take a photo of your 'why' and use it as your phone's lock screen
- Write your top three reasons for losing weight and put them where you can see them every day – on the bathroom mirror, the fridge door (and maybe in the fridge), the car dashboard, in your day planner or on a recipe book stand that can move around with you

2. **Wear them**
   - Design and print an inspirational t-shirt that tugs at your conscious mind every time you wear it.

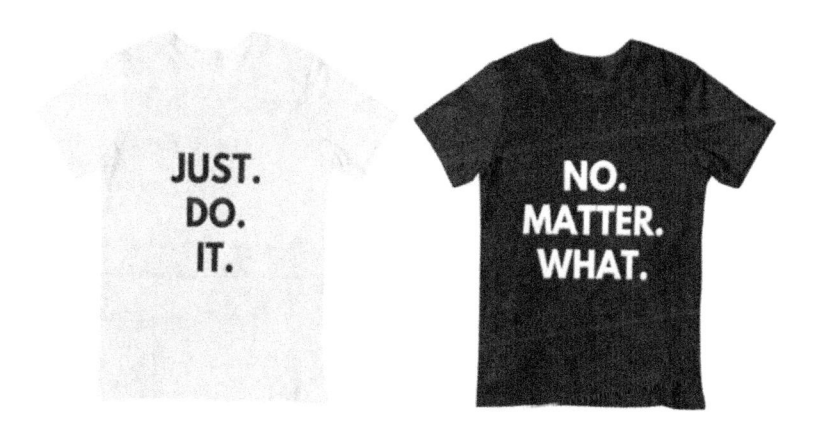

✓ Include inspirational quotes in your day

Inspirational quotes can create subliminal messages that excite and motivate you, and speak to your commitment and determination. Look out for ones that are heartfelt and truly resonate with you, then keep them nearby.

Some oldies but goldies…

> "I choose to make the rest of my life the best of my life." **Louise Hay**

> "Look at everything as though you were seeing it either for the first or last time. Then your time on earth will be filled with glory." **Betty Smith**

> "Life is not measured by the number of breaths we take, but by the moments that take our breath away." **Maya Angelou**

> "It's a beautiful, beautiful thing, the sun comes up, I'm having a good day." **Leigh Coldrey**

✅ "Well done you"

Reward yourself along the way. Sure, the big payoff is at the end when you are a healthy weight and feeling fabulous again – but give yourself some smaller rewards (this will help to keep you motivated).

Maybe buy new underwear (a smaller size of course), have a massage or a pedicure (anything but a food reward – after all, you're not a dog!).

✅ Keep eyes on yourself

'Watching eyes' can help you focus and self-regulate because you feel you are being observed.
- Take a photo of your eyes, then print and display it where you can see your eyes looking back at you when you have to make decisions that can impact your weight loss

Step 3: Stay on Track (& Conquer Your Inner Voice)

- See yourself in a mirror when you are eating in order to view yourself objectively and enhance your self-awareness
- Invest in a full-length mirror, and use it for inspiration

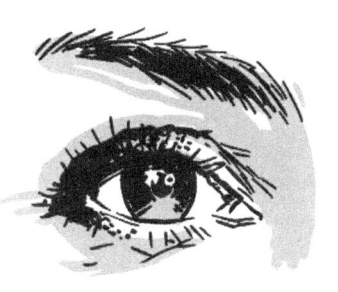

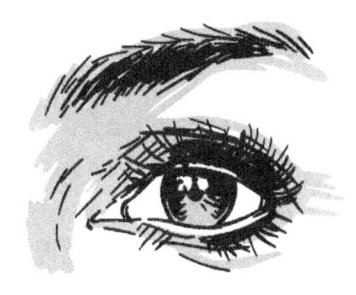

✅ Face up to yourself

Create a life-size cardboard display of yourself and stand it in your bedroom so you can step back, look at yourself and stay motivated.

✅ Visualize it, then believe it

Use visualization to generate powerful thoughts and feelings of yourself being what you want to be, and being it right now.

To do this, you need to:
- Decide want you want
- Believe you deserve it
- Be passionate about it
- Expect you will achieve it

Then,
- Create a picture or, better still, a short mental movie in your mind

Fat, Frumpy & Over 50

- Experience it with all your senses – see it, smell it, taste it, hear it, *feel it*
- Take in how motivated you are making healthy food choices right now and how easy it is
- Feel what it is like to be a healthy weight and what you are now able to do
- Mind rehearse this scenario for at least five minutes in the morning and at the end of every day before you go to sleep
- Go back through your day and look for any moments that you feel were negative or disappointing, then replay them over in your mind the way you wanted them to go

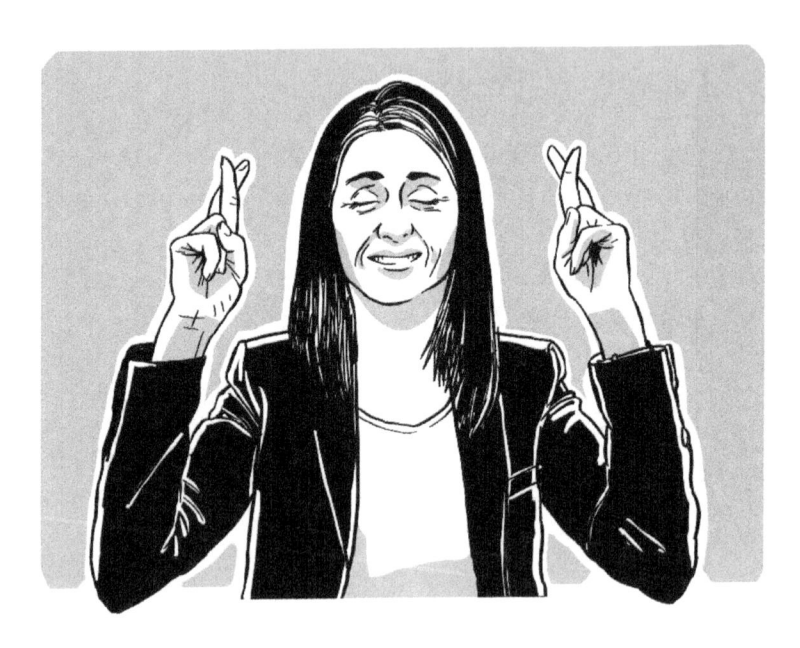

Visualize it, then believe it

Step 3: Stay on Track (& Conquer Your Inner Voice)

✓ Make sure you dress the part

What you wear really does matter. There is such a thing as 'enclothed cognition' where your clothing has an effect on the way you think, feel and function.

'Dopamine dressing' is dressing to boost your mood. By wearing a certain color, texture, or style, it is thought you can activate the release of dopamine (your feel-good chemical).

As you start out on your weight-loss journey, you may be feeling frumpy, but think about changing your style anyway and 'dress yourself healthier'.

And this includes having stylish, comfortable exercise gear to really motivate you, so have at least three outfits on hand.

✓ Write an advice column to yourself

Whatever your challenges are, write them down.
1. Describe in detail what you want help with.
2. Take your time and provide your own objective answers.

You'll see that every challenge has a solution.

✓ Listen to a message from yourself

Remember that a person's name is to that person the sweetest and most important sound in any language.
Dale Carnegie

Record an audio message to yourself on your phone.
- Use your name, talk about your purpose, your goals and include simple words of encouragement

- To connect your present and future self, listen to your message every day

✓ Stand back, and look at yourself as if you are someone else

Get a different perspective of yourself. What needs to be done seems so much more obvious when you're looking at someone else.

So, be your own adviser.
1. Imagine your current situation is somebody else's.
2. Give her a name (it helps).
3. Next 'ask' her where she is now, what her frustrations are, and what she wants to have achieved in, say, three months from now (no longer than that).
4. Finally, tell her what to do to reach her goals.

✓ Talk out loud to yourself

Talking out loud to yourself can motivate you, help you to stay focused and to resist self-criticism.
- Say your affirmations out loud every day
- Talk encouragingly to yourself as you look in the mirror

> *Only you can allow yourself to explore the person in the mirror.*
> *Only you can coax yourself into a daring adventure to find your untapped potential.*
> **Vironika Tugaleva,**
> **The Art of Talking to Yourself**

✓ Think about someone you care about having the same thoughts as you

Think of yourself as a relative, friend or co-worker who you don't want to let down.

What thoughtful, positive advice would you want to give to them (then give that advice to yourself)?

✓ Listen to motivational speakers

Have you ever watched a TED Talk on YouTube with the intention of simply passing time, but ended up with a surge of motivation to do something? Or maybe you've sat in on an in-person speech that actually inspired you when really you thought it was going to be something that you just had to patiently sit through?

Well, if you have, then you understand what motivational speeches are and how they can have a positive impact on you.

Do your own research to find and watch the ones that really focus on wellbeing and energize you to take action to get this weight-loss thing done.

✓ Make a happy place at home and work

By creating positive, happy places that bring you joy you'll make it easier to sustain a positive, open mindset.
- Make a space where you can gather your thoughts, spend time by yourself and recharge
- Display items that connect with good memories and strong, positive feelings around your home
- Let the sunshine in
- Add fresh flowers or plants to lift your mood

✓ Put together a music playlist that uplifts, excites and inspires you

Music has a way of imbedding itself in your memories – you make associations with music that later bring up certain experiences or states of mind. It can put your brain into a feelgood state and drown out the noise of resistance. Music holds the promise of something better.

- Create a go-to playlist of music that makes your heart sing until you feel an explosion of energy, optimism and abandon
- Tailor your music to what you want to achieve, put on your headphones and listen as it inspires you to create the momentum to stick to your goals

Search on Google or Spotify for music themes such as 'uplifting', 'motivating', 'inspiring', etc. (and don't forget about the potential thrill of classical music).

✓ Also think of movie scenes and the music scores that inspire you

Think of scenes from movies you love, that always evoke strong positive emotions in you – and can even make you sing – then think of the music embedded in those scenes. Associate the music with those exhilarating feelings and add it to your playlist, ready to use when you need to get yourself back on track.

✓ Hypnotherapy

Hypnotherapy (and guided imagery) may help you make healthier food choices and reduce food cravings as part of a weight-loss plan.

You could see a hypnotherapy practitioner, or 'do it yourself'. There are a range of 'self-hypnosis for weight loss' audio books and apps available online, many free.

Tips for improving self-hypnosis:
- Make suggestions positive and realistic
- Avoid over-ambitious suggestions such as "I will lose 10 pounds in two weeks" – instead focus on smaller, realistic goals and action steps
- Schedule time for self-hypnosis – it can be performed at any time – either during the day, or at night before you go to sleep
- Stick at it – it can take time to learn self-hypnosis but with practice, you will more quickly enter a state of deep relaxation.

✅ Acupuncture for weight loss

It is thought acupuncture (the traditional Chinese medical practice of stimulating specific points on the body, primarily by inserting very thin needles through the skin) relaxes the nervous system so it can assist with the metabolization of food, stabilize and send accurate hunger signals, and improve digestion.

You may want to consider it as part of a holistic approach to weight loss.

✅ Crystals

Advocates use crystals in their belief they are effective for weight loss, and feel motivated by them.

Choose crystals that have special significance to you and keep them nearby when you are eating.

Popular Crystals for Weight Loss		
Blue Apatite	Amethyst	Picasso Marble
Peridot	White Quartz	Gaspeite
Carnelian	Steatite	Diaspore
Peridot	Epidote	Iolite
Goldstone	Sunstone	Selenite

✓ Personal trainer

Is it time to turn to a professional?

The benefit of a personal trainer is that they can support you to maintain your behavior change, and therefore your weight-loss goals.

Working with a personal trainer can help keep you motivated, and hold you accountable to someone else.

✓ Life coach

A life coach can 'stand on the sidelines' encouraging you to reflect on, discover and achieve your personal goals.

Life coaching is forward-thinking and future-focused.

✓ Cognitive behavior therapy (CBT)

CBT is a therapeutic approach that focuses on identifying thoughts, feelings and behaviors that can be negative, unhealthy, self-limiting or unsupportive, then teaches you how to change them.

CBT can be undertaken with a therapist, however there are also several self-help books and internet-based treatment programs available.

Step 3: Stay on Track (& Conquer Your Inner Voice)

THE COGNITIVE MODEL

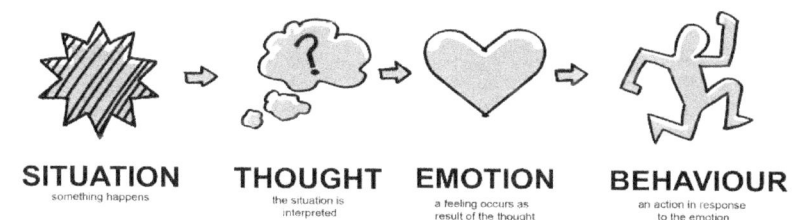

SITUATION
something happens

THOUGHT
the situation is interpreted

EMOTION
a feeling occurs as result of the thought

BEHAVIOUR
an action in response to the emotion

✓ Mindset coach

A mindset coach can help you to 'rewire' your mindset, allowing you to 'be the very best version of yourself'.

The core approach is that you already have everything you need within you to create whatever you want in your life.

✓ Psychologist

As you well know, eating is a common coping mechanism. A major aspect of weight control involves understanding and then managing your food-related challenges.

Psychologists can help you to shift your thoughts and behaviors towards building a healthy relationship with food.

Part 2: <u>Crush</u> your diet-crashing cravings <u>in-the-moment</u> if they've got you in their grip

So here it is, even with all your preparation to avoid going into the 'danger zone', the trigger has been pulled, you're indulging in negative self-talk, and you're feeling that overwhelming urge to give in to that craving.

There's no way around it – the first thing you must do is just stop, even for a moment. Every break in this cycle will always begin with that one strong-willed decision to respond differently this time.

It will pass, *if you let it*. You must believe that, regardless of how deep and forceful the craving is, you can get beyond it. Each craving has an expiration – most last about two minutes and are satisfied by about four bites – and if you don't respond to it, after a period of time, it will go away.

So, in that moment when you're on the precipice of giving in, use all your senses to redirect your thoughts by engaging your mind (mental distractions), your body (physical distractions) and your emotions. And get busy thinking, doing or feeling something else.

Here's how to do it…

✅ Just breathe

When you are stressed, your breathing is shallow, your breaths are small, and you use your upper chest and shoulders to breathe instead of your diaphragm. You also tend to experience more cravings.

Deliberately controlling your breathing pattern, with the aim of reducing stress, will help you to instantly relax, increase your feeling of calmness and effectively reduce your overwhelming craving.

To get you started:
1. Stand up (get out of your chair if you're sitting down) and straighten your shoulders.
2. Become aware of your breathing.
3. Take a deep breath, yawn, blink a few times, roll your eyes in a big circle slowly clockwise, and then anti-clockwise.
4. As you breathe in and out, hold onto a loving memory or thought.
5. Now, as you continue, choose one of the following controlled breathing techniques.

Diaphragmatic/'Belly Breathing' (Lying Down)
1. Lie on your back on a flat surface (or on your bed) with your knees bent. Use a pillow under your head and knees for support if that's more comfortable.
2. Place one hand on your chest and the other on your belly, just below your rib cage.
3. Breathe in slowly through your nose, letting the air in deeply, towards your lower belly. The hand on your belly should rise.
4. Tighten your abdominal muscles and let them fall inward as you exhale through pursed lips. The hand on your belly should move down to its original position.

Diaphragmatic/'Belly Breathing' (Sitting)
1. Sit comfortably with your knees bent and your shoulders, head, and neck relaxed.
2. Place one hand on your chest and the other just below your rib cage.

Step 3: Stay on Track (& Conquer Your Inner Voice)

3. Breathe in slowly through your nose so that your stomach moves outwards against your hand. The hand on your chest should remain as still as possible throughout the breath.
4. Tighten your stomach muscles, letting them fall inward as you exhale through pursed lips so that your stomach moves inwards against your hand. The hand on your chest should remain as still as possible.

4-6-8 'Relaxing Breath' Technique

1. Place the tip of your tongue against the roof of your mouth, directly behind your upper front teeth, and keep it there throughout the entire exercise.
2. Exhale through your mouth, making a 'whoosh' sound out loud.
3. Close your mouth and inhale silently through your nose for a count of four.
4. Hold the breath for a count of six.
5. Exhale through your mouth again, making a 'whoosh' sound for a count of eight.

✓ Ride it out

Use this one-minute trick straight away to stop yourself giving into that craving.

1. Ride (and count) it out… one minute at a time (or 10 seconds, five seconds or even one second if that's what it takes).
2. Live with the momentary discomfort, knowing your craving is from an emotional trigger, is not physiological, and that it will soon pass.
3. Have a logical argument with yourself… tell yourself you are stronger than your craving.
4. Dig your heels in and refuse to crumble.

5. Say "I *don't* eat that" (instead of "I *can't* eat that") and remind yourself that you've got this.

✅ Surf the wave

Cravings are like waves that rise, build to a peak, and then fall. 'Urge surfing' is a mindful way to conquer them.

Here's what to do…
1. Use your breathing to let your craving build, and then crash as you breathe out.
2. Recognize what you are feeling right now. Are you agitated, bored, lonely? Is your body tense?
3. Be curious about your craving, notice the sensation, allow it to be there, sit with it, allow it to wash over you and then go into shore. Go with the wave instead of swimming against it, and your craving will wash away.

✅ Stretch your body

Stretching acts as a physical distraction – helping you to wait it out while your craving passes.

If you're sitting:
- Raise your legs and tense your muscles
- Press your feet into floor
- Press your arms into the side of the chair
- Push your shoulders into the top of the chair

If you're standing:
- Stretch your arms behind your back and clasp your hands together
- Stand on your tip toes then crouch down slightly
- Press your palms together in front of you
- Flex your chest muscles

Step 3: Stay on Track (& Conquer Your Inner Voice)

- Join your hands behind your head and stretch your elbows backwards

✅ Touch your lips

Your lips, especially the upper lip, are full of sensory nerve endings, making them sensitive to the touch.

Lightly brushing two fingers over your lips will give you a wave of calm, helping you refocus, feel comforted and rapidly lose interest in that craving.

You could also put on some lip salve as a further, comforting distraction so you'll have even less interest in mindless eating.

✅ Yoga techniques to keep you on track

When that craving is chasing you down, you are probably holding stress in your jaw. The 'Lions Breath' yoga move (below) can help to loosen your jaw, release stress and allow your craving to pass.

1. Inhale through your nose.
2. On the exhale, stick out your tongue, pointing it down to your chin, and raise your eyes.
3. Repeat 5 times.

The yoga technique of humming like a bumble bee (below) can also calm you down and give you time to refocus.

1. Sit upright in a chair or lie on your bed. Close your eyes and mouth, keeping your teeth slightly apart.
2. Breath in deeply through your nose, then breath out through your nose, keeping your lips closed but not pursed and making a humming sound as you do so. Keep the hum going until you've completely exhaled.
3. Repeat 5 times.

✅ Touch your forehead

You've probably used the kinesiology emotional stress release technique without realizing it when you've been anxious. It's thought to help attract blood to the frontal lobe of your brain, responsible for reasoning, and has a calming effect.

So, try using the tips of your fingers to touch two points on your forehead, about halfway between your eyebrows and hairline. Let the palms of your hands rest lightly on your closed eyes and your cheeks. It's the classic "I'm thinking" pose, and a great distraction from your craving.

✅ Chant

Chanting can decrease stress and anxiety as well as increase positive mood, feelings of relaxation and focused attention (regardless of the tradition or belief system involved in the chanting practice).

- In a craving crisis, *immediately* repeat a vocal chantra (either your own or the universal "om") to re-focus your mind
- Repeat the chantra for as long as you need to for the craving to pass

✅ Acupressure

Auricular acupressure may be effective in reducing stress, improving metabolism and boosting digestion.

While acupuncture uses needles to stimulate specific points around the body, acupressure is done by stimulating these points through massage therapy. It will give you something else to focus on.

Step 3: Stay on Track (& Conquer Your Inner Voice)

Here's how to do it:
1. Place the tips of your index fingers right in front of your ears, next to the fleshy bump above the earlobe.
2. Massage for 30 to 60 seconds.

✅ Get into a relaxed state of mind

Cultivating a more restful, relaxed state of mind can support you to be more resilient in the face of challenges.

See how you go with this technique:
1. Sit or lie down somewhere and close your eyes.
2. Picture a movie projection screen in front of your forehead and on the screen is a big number '1'. Imagine as you breathe in slowly through your nose, the number '1' is drawn closer until it sticks to your forehead.
3. Then release that breath, slowly, and imagine that as you breathe out, the number '1' slides down through your face and is blown out by your mouth.
4. Now see the number '2' on your screen in front of you. Repeat the same as for number '1', remembering to breathe deeply and slowly, in through your nose and out through your mouth.
5. Repeat until you reach the number '20'.

✅ Use a mantra to practice your 'active no'

A mantra will help you ride the emotional upswings and push you through the downswings.

Rehearse a simple mantra, in your mind or out loud, so you know it off by heart and it's easily recalled when you need it.

It could be, "Whatever happens right now, I am not going to [fill in your blank]."

✓ Wash your hands in warm water

Removing yourself from what is tempting you to wash your hands can initiate 'psychological separation' from your current craving and give you time to regain your inner strength.

✓ The healing light exercise

Pure light visualization is another relaxation technique. It revolves around the idea of absorbing positive and getting rid of negative energy. It gives you another effective distraction.

1. Sit or lie down, get comfortable and close your eyes.
2. Choose a color that you find most soothing and relaxing.
3. Focus on your breathing and begin to breathe slowly.
4. Now imagine that there is a light above your head, and that it is your soothing and relaxing color. Every time you breathe in some of this light washes over you.
5. Imagine that everywhere the light touches, it soothes and relaxes you. Every time you breathe in, more and more light washes over you. It washes over your head, eyes, jaw and neck, continuing to sooth and relax you. More and more light then washes over you until it has touched all of your body.
6. Remember that the light comes from an endless source, and the more light you breathe in, the more light is available. Keep breathing in more and more light, more and more... more and more.

✓ The Sedona Method will get you unstuck

The Sedona Method is a simple technique that shows you how to take control and let go of any painful or unwanted feelings *in the moment*.

Step 3: Stay on Track (& Conquer Your Inner Voice)

1. Describe the emotion behind your craving (for example, frustration, anxiety, boredom, etc.). What does it *look* like? How *big* is it? What *color* is it?
2. Put your hand on where the emotion sits in your body.
3. Ask yourself if you were given the opportunity to let this feeling go, *could* you?
4. Ask yourself if you were given the opportunity to let this feeling go, *would* you?
5. If you would let it go, when?
6. Use a symbolic way (for example, blowing on your hands) to let go of that feeling.
7. Use another symbolic way (for example, grasping your hands) to fill the vacuum and replace the old feeling with a new uplifting one.
8. Repeat this process until you are feeling positive and you've left that craving behind.

✅ When you think about quitting, instead think about why you started

Always keep your 'why' and goals close by, and *immediately* sit down and *thoughtfully* read your reasons for wanting to be a healthy weight, and the goals you have committed to. Feel them, visualize them, remember how important they are to you in this moment.

✅ Use numbers to pull your thoughts back

Even if you aren't a math person, numbers can help distract and re-center you.

Try:
- Running through a times table in your head
- Counting forwards by threes (1, 4, 7, 10 and so on)

- Counting backwards from 100
- Choosing a number and thinking of five ways you could make the number (6 + 11 = 17, 20 − 3 = 17, 8 × 2 + 1 = 17, etc.)

✅ Describe what's around you

- Spend a few minutes taking in your surroundings and noting what you see. Use all of your five senses to provide as much detail as possible (such as, "this bench is red, but the bench over there is green")
- Describe (out loud) the features of the room you are in and draw it in your mind as you say it
- Look at an object close to you (maybe a piece of fruit) and guess what it feels like, smells like, etc.

✅ Give yourself some serotonin-boosting self-care

Self-care is doing something that nurtures or honors yourself.

When your inner strength is waning, self-care can help build up your resilience.

In-the-moment
- Brush your hair (or your teeth)
- Shake and wiggle your body
- Smile!

When you have 5 minutes
- Go through the calming, methodical process of brewing and pouring tea (and sit to drink it)
- Text a friend
- Look at old photos
- Have your own private dance party

Step 3: Stay on Track (& Conquer Your Inner Voice)

When you have 15 minutes
- Have a long, hot shower
- Water the plants in your garden
- Have a cat nap
- Phone someone you love

When you have an hour or more
- Watch a competitive quiz show
- Soak in a hot bath
- Do a workout or join an on-line yoga class
- Get a massage
- Read a book
- Binge watch a series on a streaming service

✓ Make up lists in your mind to grab back your focus

- Think about lists, in alphabetical order, of whatever comes to mind (fruit, women's names, countries, etc.)
- Notice sights, sounds, smells, tastes and things you are touching, name them then let them go
- Use the 5-4-3-2-1 tool to name five things you can see, four things you can physically feel, three things you can hear, two things you can smell, and one thing you can taste

✓ Make yourself laugh

Laughter increases the feel-good endorphins that are released by your brain, as well as activating and relieving your stress response.
- Read some silly jokes
- Watch a funny YouTube cat video, a comedian or a TV show you enjoy

✅ Go straight to your music playlist

Choose uplifting music from your playlist to instantly put your brain into a pleasurable state and drown out the noise of your craving. Sing along, and out loud.

Or sing a line from your favourite song over and over (this will access your flow state and sense of wellbeing).

✅ Sit down and write a gratitude list

Being grateful helps you to settle and be less reactive. It is in this calm state that you can make heathier choices about your eating.

Always begin with the words, "I am grateful". For instance, it could be "I am grateful to be able to recognize and understand my food triggers".

Even if you aren't feeling overly positive about your weight on a particular day, try and find something to be grateful for.

The more positives you can find, the more likely you will be to stick to your healthy weight goals.

✅ Engage your strongest human sense – your sense of smell

One of the quickest ways to stamp out your cravings is to engage one or more of your senses – sight, sound, taste, smell, touch. But with five senses to choose from, which one trumps the rest?

Smell is in fact the strongest human sense. Your olfactory receptor neurons, which are located behind your sinuses, are the only neurons in your body that are exposed to air. They make physical contact with whatever molecules make up an odor, instantly sending that information to your brain.

Because these receptors are so close physically to your hippocampus and amygdala (which is a huge factor in memory retention), smell is considered the strongest and quickest memory inducer, affecting emotion and making it the biggest nostalgia and behavior catalyst of the sensory bunch.

Think of smells that trigger life-affirming memories for you, then seek them out when you need some positive reinforcement. Use them on your skin or clothes, in the air, on your bedsheets, etc.

Essential oils

Aromatherapy, or breathing in the scent of essential oils (distilled and pressed from aromatic plants), may calm your mind and curb your food cravings, especially for sugar.

They can be used in different ways including warmed in a diffuser or added to carrier oils then massaged onto your skin. Essential oils can be used individually or blended together.

Essential Oils for Weight Loss		
Sage	Juniper	Ginger
Lemon	Cinnamon	Fennel
Lavender	Bergamot	Lemongrass

✅ Put on your go-to positive symbol

Wearing something to 'decorate' yourself is a form of self-expression that can change how you see yourself and how you feel. Whether it is a statement piece of jewelry, a designer scarf, or maybe red lipstick, what you choose can reflect who you are and how you want to present yourself to the world.

How can it change the way you see yourself or how you feel? It could be that wearing a certain piece of jewelry makes you feel empowered. Or that certain objects hold wonderful, positive memories for you. Or it could be that you just love the look of Dior's 'Rouge Dior Couture Finish' lipstick.

It's such a personal thing. So, put on your go-to positive symbol, and shove those tempting, negative thoughts away.

✅ Go straight to your 'buzz list', the everyday wins that leave you smiling

Write a list of the everyday things you like to do, and people, places or objects that make you smile. Then, when your resistance is plummeting, do something from your list and give yourself a 'happy' boost and crush that craving.

Think about…
- Bursting some bubble wrap
- Smelling some fresh, sun-dried bedsheets
- Gulping that first mouthful of water (when you're the thirstiest you've ever been in your life)
- Squeezing a huge blackhead (on someone else!)
- Staring at the brightness of the full moon
- Doing something for someone else that makes both of you smile

✅ Listen to a mood-boosting podcast

Right now, it's all about distracting yourself from that craving that is raging through your mind. What could be better than a podcast that you can access at any time, listen to on-the-go, and all while gaining insight into some of the world's most brilliant minds, fascinating events and inspirational stories.

So, get those headphones on and start listening to a reeaallly good podcast series where you can't wait for the next episode.

✅ Watch your favorite movie scene

What's 'that' movie scene that pulls at your heartstrings and makes the world stop for a while. When you need a shot of pure joy, escape into the warm embrace of your favorite feel-good movie – the one that will leave you feeling happy and in a positive mindset.

Get lost in it, lift your emotions, and let your craving pass.

✅ Have a quick go-to list of foods you can eat in a craving crisis

Go-to-foods	Calories
1 cup air-popped popcorn	31
1 hard-boiled egg	78
1 medium carrot + 2 tablespoons hummus	100
1 cup broth-based or pureed vegetable soup	100
15 medium strawberries	100
3 wholegrain crackers + 1 slice low-fat cheese	100
14 raw almonds or 20 pistachios	100
½ cup edamame beans	105
1 cup sugar-free hot chocolate with skim milk	137
½ cup toasted pumpkin seeds	143
3 wholegrain crackers + tinned tuna in water	160
4-5 squares dark chocolate (70% to 90%)	170
1 small apple + 1 tablespoon peanut butter	172

✅ Keep your hands busy

One simple action to stop yourself giving into that craving is to hold an object in your hands – preferably something that requires both hands – or you could squeeze a couple of stress balls. Try twiddling some worry beads or do something rewarding such as knitting, drawing, writing, etc.

Do anything that will keep your hands occupied for a while. This will not only provide an instant distraction but will actually prevent you from physically reaching for that unhealthy food that is calling out, "Yoohoo, I'm here!".

✅ Play a digital game

Playing digital games with a high degree of optical stimulation (like Tetris) can distract your visual working memory allowing images of food to go away.

✅ Tap away your cravings

Emotional freedom technique (EFT), or 'tapping', is thought to release negative emotions caused by disruptions to your body's natural energy flow. The basic EFT procedure involves tapping lightly but firmly, using both your index and middle finger, on eight points of your body:
- beginning of your eyebrow (by the top your nose)
- side of your eye
- under your eye
- under your nose
- your chin
- your collarbone
- under your arm
- top of your head

Step 3: Stay on Track (& Conquer Your Inner Voice)

Before you start tapping, choose a positive statement that empowers you and keep saying it either in your mind or out loud as you tap each point.

For example, your statement could be, "Even though I feel stressed and crave chocolate right now, I believe in myself and my ability to succeed".

At the very least, by trying EFT, you'll distract yourself long enough to allow time for the craving to pass.

✅ Pat, play with or cuddle your dog, cat, rabbit... (or grandchildren?)

Many people believe dogs (and cats?) are a necessary ingredient in our emotional well-being. When a dog puts their head on your lap, it can instantly calm you.

So, distract yourself with whatever (friendly) animal is nearby. By focusing on them, you'll stop focusing on yourself.

✅ If you don't have a cute animal nearby, look instead at photos of them

This will light up the pleasure centers in your brain and make you instantly happier (while also distracting you).

When parents look at their baby and their baby stares into their eyes, even though the baby can't talk, parents get an oxytocin boost just by eye contact.

Animals have somehow hijacked this bonding pathway just by making eye contact with you. Look at photos of your own dog or cat if you can (for the strongest emotional pull), or find random ones on the internet. Just make sure they are looking directly at you.

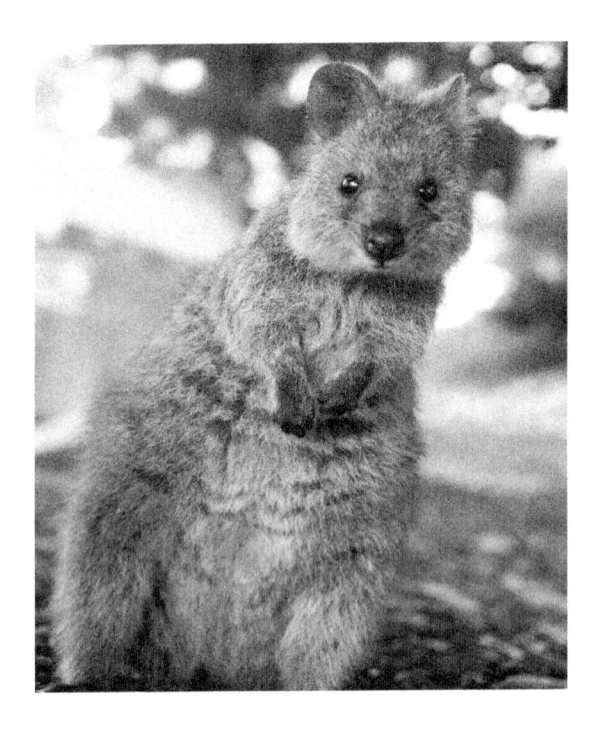

✅ Plan a holiday

Simply planning a trip, or at least thinking about it, can help boost happiness and alleviate stress. It can also pull you out of the current moment – with its challenge of sending you into a craving crisis – and get you back to being goal-focused.

Booking (and anticipating) a trip – even just getting it on the calendar – might be just what you need to ride this craving out.

✅ Get outside

When you get caught up in the moment, and stop focusing on your healthy weight goals, it can help to plant your feet outside and get yourself inspired again.

Step 3: Stay on Track (& Conquer Your Inner Voice)

Go for a bushwalk (if you can), take your dog for a long walk (they will thank you for it) or just go for a short stroll if that's all the time you have. And maybe take your shoes off? Get some fresh air. Get some sunshine. The important thing is to break into whatever challenging thoughts you have in this moment and quickly change the environment around you. So, step outside and let it give you the boost you need.

And if you can't get outside… have a poster on your wall, or a photo you keep with you, of a beach, a lake, the ocean, a forest, the night sky, or whatever is your favorite place, then *immerse yourself in it and smile*. There are also plenty of apps and downloads of nature sounds to listen to. Just search the internet for 'sounds from nature relaxing apps' or similar.

✅ Remind yourself that you are the fabulous person your dog thinks you are

And last, but not least… live up to your dog's absolute belief in you!

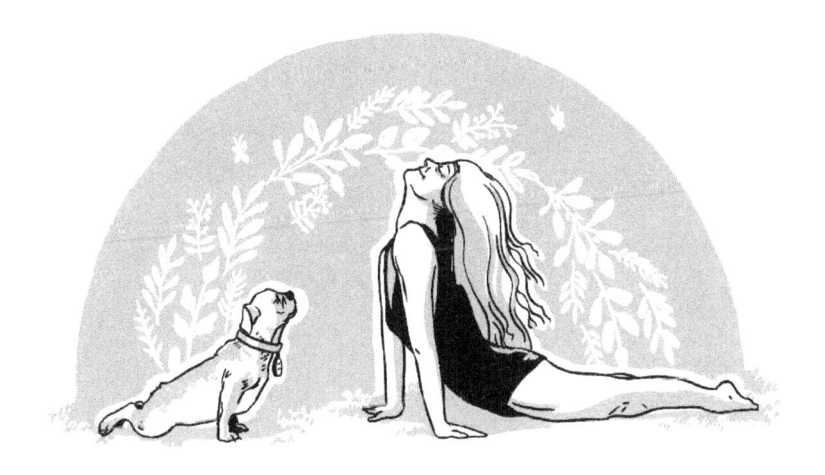

Conclusion

So, there you have it. I hope you've enjoyed reading this book and that exploring some of the practical tips, tools and strategies have been helpful for you on your weight-loss journey.

My intention in writing this book is to empower you to consistently make food choices that align with what matters most to you. And, importantly, to remind you that you are worth it.

It is my sincere wish that:
- You no longer take for granted you will always have time to put it off until later
- You realize you have one life to live and you're not prepared to let another day slip away
- You know feeling fabulous makes you happier than eating chocolate cake!

Congratulations, and pat yourself on the back.

You go girl!

And one final thing...

I'd love to hear from you about your own experiences and if this book has been helpful. What did you like about it? Were there things that could have been done better? Did I miss anything that you would have liked to have seen included?

You can drop me a line or ask questions by emailing me at:

hello@jacquelinelapton.com

I'd also really appreciate it if you would review this book on Amazon.

Thank you.

Printed in Great Britain
by Amazon